RHEUMATOID ARTHRITIS:
YOUR MEDICATION EXPLAINED

MARY-CLAIRE MASON is a freelance journalist with a special interest in health. She is a member of the Medical Journalists' Association and the Guild of Health Writers. She has written for the national press, as well as for women's magazines such as *Bella*, *Woman's Realm* and *Essentials*. She is the author of the Sheldon Press book *Coping with Fibroids*. She lives in London with her husband, two cats and a Dalmatian.

DR ELAINE SMITH was a rheumatologist at Guy's Hospital, London. She currently works as a general physician at a hospital in New South Wales, Australia, where she has also set up a rheumatology service. She is on the editorial board of the *Drug and Therapeutics Bulletin*, published by the Consumers' Association.

C000163599

Overcoming Common Problems Series

For a full list of titles please contact
Sheldon Press, Marylebone Road, London NW1 4DU

Antioxidants
DR ROBERT YOUNGSON

The Assertiveness Workbook
A plan for busy women
JOANNA GUTMANN

Beating the Comfort Trap
DR WINDY DRYDEN AND JACK
GORDON

Body Language
How to read others' thoughts by their
gestures
ALLAN PEASE

Body Language in Relationships
DAVID COHEN

Calm Down
How to cope with frustration and anger
DR PAUL HAUCK

Cancer – A Family Affair
NEVILLE SHONE

The Cancer Guide for Men
HELEN BEARE AND NEIL PRIDDY

The Candida Diet Book
KAREN BRODY

Caring for Your Elderly Parent
JULIA BURTON-JONES

Cider Vinegar
MARGARET HILLS

Comfort for Depression
JANET HORWOOD

Considering Adoption?
SARAH BIGGS

Coping Successfully with Hay Fever
DR ROBERT YOUNGSON

**Coping Successfully with Joint
Replacement**
DR TOM SMITH

Coping Successfully with Migraine
SUE DYSON

Coping Successfully with Pain
NEVILLE SHONE

Coping Successfully with Panic Attacks
SHIRLEY TRICKETT

Coping Successfully with PMS
KAREN EVENNETT

**Coping Successfully with Prostate
Problems**
ROSY REYNOLDS

Coping Successfully with RSI
MAGGIE BLACK AND PENNY GRAY

**Coping Successfully with Your Hiatus
Hernia**
DR TOM SMITH

**Coping Successfully with Your Irritable
Bladder**
DR JENNIFER HUNT

**Coping Successfully with Your Irritable
Bowel**
ROSEMARY NICOL

**Coping When Your Child Has Special
Needs**
SUZANNE ASKHAM

Coping with Anxiety and Depression
SHIRLEY TRICKETT

Coping with Blushing
DR ROBERT EDELMANN

Coping with Breast Cancer
DR EADIE HEYDERMAN

Coping with Bronchitis and Emphysema
DR TOM SMITH

Coping with Candida
SHIRLEY TRICKETT

Coping with Chronic Fatigue
TRUDIE CHALDER

Coping with Coeliac Disease
KAREN BRODY

Coping with Cystitis
CAROLINE CLAYTON

Coping with Depression and Elation
DR PATRICK McKEON

Coping with Eczema
DR ROBERT YOUNGSON

Coping with Endometriosis
JO MEARS

Coping with Epilepsy
FIONA MARSHALL AND
DR PAMELA CRAWFORD

Coping with Fibroids
MARY-CLAIRE MASON

Coping with Gallstones
DR JOAN GOMEZ

Coping with Headaches and Migraine
SHIRLEY TRICKETT

Coping with a Hernia
DR DAVID DELVIN

Coping with Psoriasis
PROFESSOR RONALD MARKS

Coping with Rheumatism and Arthritis
DR ROBERT YOUNGSON

Overcoming Common Problems Series

Coping with Stammering
TRUDY STEWART AND JACKIE
TURNBULL

Coping with Stomach Ulcers
DR TOM SMITH

Coping with Strokes
DR TOM SMITH

Coping with Thrush
CAROLINE CLAYTON

Coping with Thyroid Problems
DR JOAN GOMEZ

Coping with Your Cervical Smear
KAREN EVENNETT

Crunch Points for Couples
JULIA COLE

Curing Arthritis – The Drug-Free Way
MARGARET HILLS

**Curing Arthritis – More ways to a
drug-free life**
MARGARET HILLS

Curing Arthritis Diet Book
MARGARET HILLS

Curing Arthritis Exercise Book
MARGARET HILLS AND JANET
HORWOOD

Cystic Fibrosis – A Family Affair
JANE CHUMBLEY

Depression
DR PAUL HAUCK

Depression at Work
VICKY MAUD

**Everything Parents Should Know
About Drugs**
SARAH LAWSON

Feverfew
DR STEWART JOHNSON

Gambling – A Family Affair
ANGELA WILLANS

Garlic
KAREN EVENNETT

Getting a Good Night's Sleep
FIONA JOHNSTON

The Good Stress Guide
MARY HARTLEY

Heart Attacks – Prevent and Survive
DR TOM SMITH

**Helping Children Cope with Attention
Deficit Disorder**
DR PATRICIA GILBERT

Helping Children Cope with Bullying
SARAH LAWSON

Helping Children Cope with Divorce
ROSEMARY WELLS

Helping Children Cope with Dyslexia
SALLY RAYMOND

Helping Children Cope with Grief
ROSEMARY WELLS

Helping Children Cope with Stammering
JACKIE TURNBULL AND TRUDY
STEWART

Hold Your Head Up High
DR PAUL HAUCK

How to Accept Yourself
DR WINDY DRYDEN

How to Be Your Own Best Friend
DR PAUL HAUCK

How to Cope when the Going Gets Tough
DR WINDY DRYDEN AND JACK
GORDON

How to Cope with Anaemia
DR JOAN GOMEZ

How to Cope with Bulimia
DR JOAN GOMEZ

How to Cope with Difficult Parents
DR WINDY DRYDEN AND JACK
GORDON

How to Cope with Difficult People
ALAN HOUEL WITH CHRISTIAN
GODEFROY

**How to Cope with People who Drive
You Crazy**
DR PAUL HAUCK

How to Cope with Splitting Up
VERA PEIFFER

How to Cope with Stress
DR PETER TYRER

How to Enjoy Your Retirement
VICKY MAUD

How to Improve Your Confidence
DR KENNETH HAMBLY

How to Interview and Be Interviewed
MICHELE BROWN AND GYLES
BRANDRETH

How to Keep Your Cholesterol in Check
DR ROBERT POVEY

How to Love and Be Loved
DR PAUL HAUCK

How to Pass Your Driving Test
DONALD RIDLAND

How to Raise Confident Children
CAROLE BALDOCK

How to Stand up for Yourself
DR PAUL HAUCK

Overcoming Common Problems Series

How to Start a Conversation and Make Friends
DON GABOR

How to Stick to a Diet
DEBORAH STEINBERG AND
DR WINDY DRYDEN

How to Stop Worrying
DR FRANK TALLIS

How to Succeed as a Single Parent
CAROLE BALDOCK

How to Untangle Your Emotional Knots
DR WINDY DRYDEN AND JACK
GORDON

How to Write a Successful CV
JOANNA GUTMANN

Hysterectomy
SUZIE HAYMAN

The Irritable Bowel Diet Book
ROSEMARY NICOL

The Irritable Bowel Stress Book
ROSEMARY NICOL

Is HRT Right for You?
DR ANNE MACGREGOR

Jealousy
DR PAUL HAUCK

Learning to Live with Multiple Sclerosis
DR ROBERT POVEY, ROBIN DOWIE
AND GILLIAN PRETT

Living with Angina
DR TOM SMITH

Living with Asthma
DR ROBERT YOUNGSON

Living with Crohn's Disease
DR JOAN GOMEZ

Living with Diabetes
DR JOAN GOMEZ

Living with Grief
DR TONY LAKE

Living with High Blood Pressure
DR TOM SMITH

Living with Nut Allergies
KAREN EVENNETT

Living with Osteoporosis
DR JOAN GOMEZ

Living with a Stoma
DR CRAIG WHITE

Menopause
RAEWYN MACKENZIE

The Migraine Diet Book
SUE DYSON

Motor Neurone Disease – A Family Affair
DR DAVID OLIVER

Overcoming Anger
DR WINDY DRYDEN

Overcoming Anxiety
DR WINDY DRYDEN

Overcoming Guilt
DR WINDY DRYDEN

Overcoming Jealousy
DR WINDY DRYDEN

Overcoming Procrastination
DR WINDY DRYDEN

Overcoming Shame
DR WINDY DRYDEN

Overcoming Your Addictions
DR WINDY DRYDEN AND
DR WALTER MATWEYCHUK

The Parkinson's Disease Handbook
DR RICHARD GODWIN-AUSTEN

The PMS Diet Book
KAREN EVENNETT

A Positive Thought for Every Day
DR WINDY DRYDEN

Second Time Around
ANNE LOVELL

Serious Mental Illness – A Family Affair
GWEN HOWE

Sex and Relationships
ROSEMARY STONES

The Stress Workbook
JOANNA GUTMANN

The Subfertility Handbook
VIRGINIA IRONSIDE AND SARAH
BIGGS

Talking About Anorexia
How to cope with life without starving
MAROUSHKA MONRO

Talking with Confidence
DON GABOR

Ten Steps to Positive Living
DR WINDY DRYDEN

Think Your Way to Happiness
DR WINDY DRYDEN AND JACK
GORDON

The Travellers' Good Health Guide
TED LANKESTER

Understanding Obsessions and Compulsions
A self-help manual
DR FRANK TALLIS

Understanding Your Personality
Myers-Briggs and more
PATRICIA HEDGES

Overcoming Common Problems

Rheumatoid Arthritis:
Your Medication Explained

Mary-Claire Mason and
Dr Elaine Smith

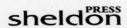

sheldon**PRESS**

Published in Great Britain in 2001
Sheldon Press
Holy Trinity Church
Marylebone Road
London NW1 4DU

British Library Cataloguing-in-Publication Data

A catalogue record for this book is available from the British Library

ISBN 0–85969–836–X

Typeset by Deltatype Limited, Birkenhead, Merseyside
Printed in Great Britain by
Biddles Ltd, *www.biddles.co.uk* Guildford and King's Lynn

Contents

1 Introduction   1
2 An Introduction to the Drugs   10
3 Painkillers and Non-steroidal Anti-inflammatory
  Drugs (NSAIDs)   21
4 Disease-modifying Anti-rheumatic Drugs (DMARDs)   30
5 Steroids   63
6 New Treatment Developments and Drug Trials   76
7 Supplements and Other Approaches   86

  Further Reading   94
  Useful Addresses   95
  Index   97

1

Introduction

Drugs play a vital part in the treatment of rheumatoid arthritis, and though at the moment there is no one drug that can cure you, the right drug treatment can let you lead a normal life. Four groups of drugs are used and it's not uncommon to be on mixed medication. Some drugs are more powerful than others, and a drug that works for one person may not necessarily work for another. Every drug can have side-effects.

So the aim of this book is to give you as much information as possible about drugs for rheumatoid arthritis so that you can understand what's on offer and get the best from your medicine.

What is rheumatoid arthritis?

'Rheumatism' is a general term for aches and pains in joints and muscles, and 'arthritis' refers to inflamed joints. A joint is where two or more bones meet and there are several types of joints that allow different degrees of movement. Some are fixed, such as the skull, some allow a little movement, such as the bones of the spine, and some are designed to allow much more movement, such as the hip, which is a ball and socket joint.

In a joint the bone surfaces are covered with smooth, slippery cartilage to reduce friction between the bones. The joint is sealed within a tough capsule lined with the synovium – a membrane that produces a lubricating fluid to keep the cartilage slippery so that the joint can move smoothly. Muscles attached to bone by tendons on either side of the joint control movement and most mobile joints have at least one bursa – a fluid-filled sac – nearby to act as a cushion at pressure points, for instance where tendons or muscles cross bones.

There are around 200 types of rheumatic disease. In the most common, osteoarthritis, the cartilage that covers the bones of the joint wears out and in severe cases the bones may rub together. Rheumatoid arthritis – the second commonest type of arthritis – affects around three in 100 people and its main feature is synovitis,

1

which is inflammation of the synovium, the joint lining. People with rheumatoid arthritis can also eventually develop what's called secondary osteoarthritis as the joint wears out.

Inflammation, the inflammatory process, is an essential way of protecting the body against injury or infection, and it's a normal part of the body's defence mechanism, the immune system.

Generally the inflammatory process ends once whatever triggered it stops. In rheumatoid arthritis, however, the inflammation persists – there's no 'off button' – and it becomes chronic and destructive.

What happens is that cells from elsewhere in the body, such as the lymph system, come to the joint and lots of cells are also produced within the joint. Some of these cells produce toxic compounds, including proteins called cytokines, which cause more inflammation (note that not all cytokines produce inflammation), which encourages more cells, and so more cytokines – a process that fuels itself.

As a result, the joint becomes swollen with excess synovial fluid and the accumulation of cells in the synovium. If the disease is not controlled, tendons and the small fluid-filled sacs (bursae) may become inflamed and, in the longer term, the capsule can stretch, which may affect the stability of the joint.

The joints often affected include the knees, toes, wrists, knuckles and middle finger joints, shoulders, hips and ankles. The neck and jaw can also be affected, but not the lower part of the back. The disease can sometimes also affect other systems in the body – for instance body secretions may dry up.

Who gets rheumatoid arthritis?

The disease affects both men and women, though women are three times more likely than men to develop it. The commonest age range for it to appear is 40–55, but it's important to stress that the disease can occur at any age and both younger and older people may develop it. Children can also be affected. Juvenile rheumatoid arthritis most often occurs between 11 and 16. Although the disease can occur in children under 11, this is rare. Children with joint problems are more likely to have some other type of arthritis, though most joint symptoms in children are often 'growing pains' and not due to arthritis at all.

Symptoms

The main symptoms include painful, stiff, swollen joints that make movement difficult, and you may feel generally unwell and off colour.

The disease can start in all sorts of ways, but the most common – known as 'insidious onset' – is for it to appear gradually over some time. Around 70 per cent of people have this sort of experience. You may start to notice early morning stiffness and discomfort in some of your joints, then notice swelling, particularly in the hands, wrists, feet and ankles, and you may feel a bit tired and possibly slightly feverish.

Less commonly, joint symptoms can occur overnight then disappear for several months but then recur. Alternatively, severe symptoms can appear almost overnight and persist. Sometimes just one joint is affected, treatment settles it down but gradually more and more joints become troublesome.

Pat's symptoms started gradually ten years ago when she was 37. 'My fingers became quite painful, but I put this down to some gardening work I'd done. The symptoms went away but then came back and then my shoulders and hips became affected and then my whole body. After about a year of trying to cope on my own I went to see the doctor.'

Jill, 64, developed the disease in her mid-thirties. 'I remember that my arms suddenly became very heavy and I had all sorts of aches and pains and I felt as though I had flu. Within three weeks I was practically paralysed. My husband had to stand me up and dress me and I was in a lot of pain.'

Sue recalls: 'I started to have problems putting on shoes, which were too tight. Then a day or two later my knees started to ache and then my hips, and within two weeks the only way I could get down the stairs was to put my back against the wall and drop one leg down at a time.'

Other symptoms
- About 30 per cent of people develop rheumatoid nodules. These painless lumps can form particularly around the elbows, backs of the heels, and around the tendons in the fingers.

- At least one in three people develop Sjogren's syndrome – a condition in which the body starts to attack the glands that produce lubricating secretions. It's a common problem and if you get this you may notice that your eyes feel dry and gritty, your mouth may become dry and women may develop a dry vagina.
- It's quite common to feel tired all the time. This could be because you're in pain and not getting a good night's sleep, but it's also likely to happen because you're anaemic. This is a common problem for people who have rheumatoid arthritis.

  Blood transports vital supplies of oxygen to body tissue but when you're anaemic, the concentration of haemoglobin – the oxygen-carrying pigment in the red blood cells – is below normal levels. There may be various reasons for this, but it's very common to become anaemic if you have a chronic illness. The production of the red blood cells in the bone marrow may be affected in some way or some of the drug treatments may mean you lose a bit of blood from the gut without knowing it. Some of the drugs known as disease-modifying anti-rheumatic drugs can reduce the bone marrow's ability to make red blood cells.
- Carpal tunnel syndrome is quite a common problem that can happen later on in the course of the disease. Numbness and tingling in the fingers may occur because the inflamed joint lining puts pressure on the median nerve where it passes into the hand via a gap called the carpal tunnel at the front of the wrist.
- Vasculitis – which is inflammation of the blood vessels – affects between 2 and 5 per cent of rheumatoid arthritis sufferers. It can cause damage to the lining of the blood vessels and make it more difficult for blood to circulate so that tissue supplied by the blood vessels can become damaged or die because of the lack of blood.
- Fluid (effusions) around the heart or lungs can occur, though, like vasculitis, this is not common.

The way that the disease affects each person is very variable, but you may be frustrated and depressed and lose confidence if you can no longer do things you previously did.

What causes rheumatoid arthritis?

It's unclear what causes the disease, but it's known as an autoimmune disease. This means that the body's immune system, which is designed to protect the body, starts to attack the body for some unknown reason.

- Stress may play a role. There's no evidence that stress causes the disease, but it may worsen it and possibly trigger a flare-up. Jill's experience is that 'emotional problems and financial worries play a big part in my disease. Stress definitely makes my symptoms worse and I have to try and keep it under control.'
- Hormones seem to influence the disease in some way. For instance, it often develops during the run-up to the menopause when women are going through a time of hormonal change (the chances of developing it are around 3 per cent for women aged 45 – see next point on genetics for general risk) and many women find that they feel much better when hormone levels are high during pregnancy.
- Genetic make-up has some part to play. There is a slightly increased risk in some families, but this is not strong. It is more the case that you inherit genes that give you a slightly greater chance of developing the disease, which, it's thought, may be triggered by some environmental factor, such as a virus, though experts are by no means certain about this. If you have no family history of the disease, your chances of developing it are thought to be around 1 per cent. However, this goes up to around 5 per cent if someone in your family has it – your brother or sister, for example – and up to around 30 per cent if you have an identical twin with the disease. So genetics are important, but only fill in one part of the picture. Other factors are involved, which is why rheumatoid arthritis is known as a multi-factorial disease.
- Diet isn't thought to cause the disease, but it's possible that certain foods may worsen symptoms once the disease has developed. Sue says, 'since my daughter was born last year I've avoided red wine as it makes my symptoms much worse.'

Diagnosis

It's not always easy or straightforward to diagnose the disease, so it's important to see a rheumatologist – a doctor who specializes in the treatment of arthritis and rheumatic diseases – to ensure a correct diagnosis is made. Aching joints are a very common symptom, but the most likely cause is a viral infection and most people with aching joints don't have rheumatoid arthritis. Powerful drugs with toxic side-effects may be used to treat the disease, so it's important to make sure that you really do have the disease before you take these drugs.

There is no single diagnostic test. Your doctor will make a diagnosis by making an overall assessment of your health based on a number of indicators. He or she will talk to you about your symptoms, carry out a clinical examination and look at various test results.

Clinical examination

This is a very important part of the assessment. Your doctor will examine your joints to look for tell-tale signs of inflammation, such as a puffy, tender joint. He or she will gently squeeze the joint to see if it aches, because this is a sign of inflammation, and look for signs of swelling and tenderness. A joint that aches because of a viral infection is usually not as obviously swollen and tender as in cases of rheumatoid arthritis. The doctor will also note how warm the joint feels as this, too, is a sign of inflammation. An inflamed joint is also likely to have a texture like bread dough, due to the thickening of the synovial membrane, whereas the joint will feel hard and knobbly in osteoarthritis.

Your doctor will also look at the pattern of joint problems in your body and will want to see how many problematical joints you have as usually more joints become affected as the disease develops. There's also normally a symmetrical pattern, joints on both sides of the body being affected.

A common pattern is for the knuckle and middle joints of the index and middle fingers on both hands to be affected. Wrists are also usually affected, as are the elbows, shoulders, hips, knees, ankles and the equivalent of the knuckles of the toes. The disease can affect the neck but rarely affects the lumbar spine (in the lower back) or thoracic spine (in the middle of the back).

The doctor will also want to know how long you've had problems. Achy joints caused by a viral infection will usually clear up within 12 weeks whereas problems persist in cases of rheumatoid arthritis. You will be asked if you have problems getting out of bed in the morning, as prolonged early morning stiffness is another feature of the condition.

Blood tests are done to look at the levels of various constituents in the blood. For instance, white blood cells are produced to fight infection, platelets are a type of blood cell that play an important part in blood clotting and haemoglobin carries oxygen in the red blood cells.

Blood tests can identify signs of inflammation. The two tests most often used are the original and best-known one, which is the ESR test (erythrocyte sedimentation rate), and the newer CRP test (C-reactive protein). Each test is as good as the other, so the one you are offered will simply depend on your doctor's preferences.

The results give information about inflammation in your body. When inflammation is present the readings are usually higher, though some people can have a higher reading but be doing well. The normal ESR range is from 1 to 15 mm/hr, and a higher reading and a higher platelet count tends to mean the disease is more active. It normally drops and the platelet count is lower when the drugs are working or when you're in remission or going through a good phase. Your ESR reading may be normal if the test is done just before the ESR levels start to rise. Some people with active disease have normal ESR levels, though this is rare. It's important to remember that the reading may also be high because of some other health problem or infection.

Your blood will also be tested for the presence of an antinuclear antibody that occurs in about 30 per cent of people who have rheumatoid arthritis. Antibodies are proteins that are produced to fight and destroy invading micro-organisms, but when an auto-immune disease is active antibodies that attack the body's own tissue may develop.

Your blood will also be checked for a protein called 'the rheumatoid factor', which occurs in the blood of about 70 to 80 per cent of people with the disease. There are some people who have this factor who don't have the disease, and some people don't have this protein at the start of the disease, however. It's not a definitive test for rheumatoid arthritis, but if you have a high level in your blood and your joints are inflamed, then you may well have the disease.

X-rays are taken to check the state of the joints and look for early warning signs of bone damage called 'erosions'. These are when the bones near (periarticular) or at the joint surface (articular) are eaten away. This underlying damage can happen silently without you necessarily being aware of it, so it's important your bones are checked by taking an X-ray. Some people have mild disease without erosions. If erosions do show up, however, your doctor is likely to advise that you need to take powerful drugs known as disease-modifying anti-rheumatic drugs to prevent further deterioration of the joints.

It's likely your hands and feet will be X-rayed even if they're not causing problems because they're a good indicator of whether you're developing erosions. This is because they are often the first places where erosions develop.

Joints suffering symptoms will also be X-rayed. A few centres are using magnetic resonance imaging (MRI) to help make an earlier diagnosis, but this option isn't widely available. MRI is a diagnostic technique that produces three-dimensional images of the structures inside the body without using X-rays or other radiation.

'Watchful waiting' may actually be the best method of diagnosis sometimes. For instance, if you have a history of aching joints, but no swelling in them and X-rays and blood tests are normal, it's likely your doctor will want to wait and see what happens. Within a year it should become clear whether or not you're going to develop the disease.

How severe is the disease?

There are no hard-and-fast rules about this disease, and it's difficult to predict how you'll be affected as time passes. You may have periods when the disease seems to flare up, you feel very unwell and are getting a lot more pain, stiffness and swelling than you normally do. There may be times, too, when it goes away and you seem to be in remission, which means you have hardly any symptoms.

It's important to keep repeating that the way in which the disease develops can be very variable. Some people will have mild problems and feel relatively unaffected by the disease, while others – perhaps 1 in 20 – will have severe problems. Equally, lots of people will be in the middle somewhere and, by looking after their joints and receiving the right drug treatment, be able to lead normal lives.

It's difficult to make any predictions about how you will be affected, but there are perhaps a couple of pointers you can use. The disease is more likely to be mild if it develops in later life – for instance, when you're over 70. It's likely to be less than mild if it develops when you're younger and in your forties or so. For instance, if you're in your forties, have high levels of rheumatoid factor in your blood, plus erosions, then the disease is likely to be severe. However, it's important to repeat once again that there are no hard-and-fast rules about this disease.

How is the disease treated?

Drugs are the mainstay of treatment for many people with rheumatoid arthritis. If a lot of joint damage occurs, surgery may be needed in the longer term to correct joint deformity or stabilize a joint or put in an artificial joint. All sorts of operations can be done – for example, to release a trapped nerve or tight tendon, remove a thickened joint lining or repair a torn tendon, remove bone to ease pain or replace a joint if it's destroyed beyond repair. There are also lots of self-help measures that you can take to protect and care for your joints, such as having a healthy, varied diet and achieving the right balance between exercise and rest.

2

An Introduction to the Drugs

Drugs play a major part in helping you feel better and protecting your joints, but it's easy to feel confused about what's on offer.

How drugs can help

Drugs can make you feel better by stopping the pain and reducing inflammation. Some types of drugs can slow down the joint damage that occurs as a result of chronic inflammation of the joint lining by suppressing the immune system.

Which drugs are used?

Four types of drugs are normally used.

Analgesics and non-steroidal anti-inflammatory drugs (NSAIDs) are the first two sorts of drugs. Analgesics, commonly called painkillers, and NSAIDs are used to treat the symptoms of pain and inflammation. If you've got the disease very mildly, it's possible you may just need these two types of drugs, but they don't actually halt the underlying disease process, which damages the bones, so most rheumatologists are keen to prescribe a more powerful sort of drug once a diagnosis of rheumatoid arthritis has been made.

This leads us to the third group – disease-modifying anti-rheumatic drugs (DMARDs). These drugs are used to stop the disease from getting progressively worse. They're not painkillers as such, but in time reduce painful symptoms by slowing or halting the underlying disease process.

DMARDs are powerful and can have potentially serious side-effects. In the past they weren't used when the disease was first diagnosed because it was thought that joint damage only occurred later on in the course of the disease. They were reserved for later use and for this reason were often referred to as second-line drugs.

However, radiological studies of the way the disease develops show that joint damage actually occurs in the first few years of the disease. As a result, rheumatologists usually recommend that these drugs are used sooner rather than later so that joints can be protected from as much damage as possible.

Steroids make up the fourth group of drugs. These powerful drugs are also used to reduce inflammation and can quickly make you feel a lot better. There's also some evidence that they can reduce joint damage.

A mix of drugs

It's quite usual to take several types of drugs together to achieve effective control of your symptoms, so don't be alarmed if you find yourself in this situation. The mix can also change over time as your symptoms wax and wane and you may also find that, after a time, a drug that once worked well for you no longer does or that you start to suffer bad side-effects.

A common mix, if you've got moderately active disease, is a painkiller to take as and when needed, a NSAID, normally taken regularly, and one or possibly more DMARD. In addition, you may need a steroid injection into a joint or muscle from time to time to help with flare-ups. If you've got severe disease, you may need painkillers, a NSAID, DMARDs and low-dose steroid tablets every day. There are no hard-and-fast rules and each person's experience is different.

Jane, 65, has had the disease for over 20 years. Currently she takes a NSAID and steroid tablets each day, which suits her well. At one point she took a NSAID plus methotrexate, which is one of the DMARDs, and a steroid. This regime worked well for her for four years until she started to get sick when she took the methotrexate.

Helen, 56, says: 'I need the drugs, though I don't always like taking them, but there's only so much pain you can put up with.' She's been through various drug combinations in the last ten years since the disease was diagnosed and is now taking painkillers, a NSAID and one of the DMARDs, but says the current mix isn't controlling her symptoms enough. 'The only time I really feel fit and well is after I have a steroid injection.'

Getting help

Information

It's normal to have questions and concerns about drug treatment, so don't worry in silence, and if you're in any doubt about anything, ask for help. Your GP may be able to advise you but usually the best source of information is the specialist rheumatology clinic. Most rheumatologists will be happy to go through your queries with you and sometimes it can be helpful to prepare a list of questions before your appointment that you can go through. It is also useful to know that the specialist nurse at the clinic usually has expert knowledge and can be very helpful, so this person is another potential source of help and information. Also, bear in mind that the doctor or nurse may need to do some research before they can answer your queries. If you're feeling very anxious and finding it hard to take in information at the moment, take along someone you trust to the appointment because they're more likely to remember what's said. The clinic will also probably have various information leaflets that you can take away.

Doctors

Your GP and rheumatologist will share your care, but your rheumatologist will normally take the lead in organizing your treatment because of their expertise in the disease. If you've got mild disease, you may only see your rheumatologist once a year for a check-up, but if you've got more severe disease, you may see your rheumatologist at perhaps four to six-monthly intervals.

It's best, if possible, to see someone you trust and have confidence in. Many people are very satisfied with the help they receive, but this is not always the case.

Jane had an uneasy relationship for some years with her doctor. 'He never took any notice of what I said – particularly my concerns about my digestive problems. In the end I got very distressed and wanted to change doctors, but I wasn't sure what to do. I spoke to the clinic nurse who arranged for me to see one of the other rheumatologists. I'd worried that I might be blacklisted, but everything was fine and I felt much better once I changed doctors. It really is very important to get on with your consultant.'

As Jane's story illustrates, it may be possible to change doctors simply by talking to the specialist rheumatology nurse or you could ask your GP for help.

Whichever doctor you see, it's important to realize that, though doctors should work along similar lines, in practice they may have slightly different ways of prescribing drugs because of their experiences with them. For instance, some doctors may think certain drugs are better than others and, if your symptoms are getting worse, some may want to increase the drug dosage while others may favour adding in another drug to help you. If you feel unhappy about your doctor's advice, then you could talk to your GP about whether or not you can have a second opinion, but bear in mind that if you go through your concerns with your rheumatologist you're very likely to sort out any problems.

If you need to talk urgently to your rheumatologist in between clinic appointments, you could try ringing the consultant's secretary and ask if the rheumatologist can contact you. Make sure you have the following information for the secretary:

- your hospital number;
- details of the drugs you take;
- the date of your last clinic appointment;
- your daytime phone number.

Alternatively, ring the clinic receptionist and ask if your appointment can be brought forward or see your GP and ask if they can get your appointment brought forward. Another option is to speak to the specialist nurse, who may be able to answer your queries.

Common concerns and questions

Questions about drugs include the following.

- How can the drug help?
- When does it start to work (some of the drugs can take up to three months or so to work)?
- What are the side-effects?
- Is the drug in tablet form (most are, but a few need to be given by injection)?

- What evidence is there that the drug works?

Ask for information leaflets on the various drugs and take your time to think things over. Ask if the drugs suggested have any particular advantages for you or why the drug is being advised, what the alternatives are, if there are particularly good drugs for the sort of problems you have.

Step-up dose

A step-up dose is used for some of the more powerful drugs. What this means is that you start on a smaller dose, which is increased over a period of time to see how well you respond to the drug. Don't be alarmed and think the drug isn't working or that there's something wrong when a step-up dose is used.

Side-effects

The side-effects of the various drugs are a common concern – many people get anxious about them. These are discussed in detail in later chapters, but it's worth highlighting here several questions to ask.

- What are the short- and long-term side-effects?
- What, if anything, can you do to lessen side-effects?

There are often ways round problems and the answer sometimes can be as simple as just reducing the drug dose. So don't suffer in silence.

When it comes to side-effects, it's a case of weighing up the benefits of the drug against its disadvantages. This isn't necessarily a clear-cut exercise. What is best for you will depend on the severity of your symptoms and how much the drug helps you versus its side-effects. For instance, with some of the DMARDs, there's a slightly increased risk of developing a lymphoma, which is a form of cancer that can develop in the lymph system (this includes the lymph glands, liver, spleen and bone marrow), but this needs to be weighed up against the benefits the drugs can give you. Make sure to follow any instructions you're given about how the drug should be taken and get used to knowing what drug dosage you're on and what the maximum daily dose is for that drug – if in doubt, ask the clinic for clarification or ask a pharmacist for advice.

Mary is wary of the drugs. 'I took methotrexate for a time but I developed very loose bowels and I became so dehydrated I ended up in hospital. I'm just taking a daily steroid tablet at the moment, but I worry about taking steroids because of what I saw happen to my father years ago when he took cortisone and became moon-faced and overweight. I don't want to take a cocktail of tablets and I want to keep my body as healthy as possible unless the pain gets too much, even though my friend says I should take more drugs to have a better quality of life.'

Drug interactions

If you're taking several drugs together, you need to be aware about drug interactions. Problems can occur, for instance, when one drug reduces absorption of another drug so that it can't work so well. If both drugs are broken down by the same organ – such as the liver – this can mean one of the drugs can become more toxic because the liver can't break it down so quickly. Always make sure your doctor knows the full range of medicines you're taking, and this includes over-the-counter medicines available from the pharmacy.

If you have a change in drug treatment for some other disorder, let your doctor know about this in case of possible drug interactions.

Unexpected effects

Don't suffer in silence and don't be frightened to mention other symptoms you may notice that you weren't warned about. For instance, if you develop a dry mouth, this can cause bad breath, but the dry mouth is likely to be linked to Sjogren's syndrome rather than to drug treatment and you'll need to be particularly careful about your dental hygiene and find out what help is available for a dry mouth. Likewise, you may develop a dry vagina, which, again, is a symptom of Sjogren's syndrome and you'll need advice about vaginal lubricants. Sjogren's can also cause you to have dry eyes. If this happens, ask your doctor about artificial tear products, such as hypromellose eye drops.

Some women worry that their periods might be affected by the DMARDs, but, normally, the drugs don't affect periods and, if anything, make them lighter.

Steroids and possibly some of the DMARDs may make you more prone to getting thrush. If this happens, you may need to change the drug or take a reduced steroid dose.

Safety checks

Safety checks are done before you go on the more powerful drugs and, once on them, you will need to have regular monitoring tests (there may be a bit of variation between clinics as to how often the tests are done). For instance, tests are done to see how the liver is coping with the drug by looking at levels of certain enzymes. These are aminotransferases (aspartate aminotransferase, known as AST, and alanine aminotransferase, known as ALT). If they are higher than normal while you are taking the drug, this could be a sign that your liver is having to work very hard to break down the drug and that the liver could possibly be overloaded. A full blood count is done to keep an eye on haemoglobin (in red blood cells) and white blood cells as well as platelets.

You'll probably be given a safety record card that lists all the drugs you're taking as well as how you're responding to them. You'll be asked to note down any skin rashes or itching that you may develop as well as other symptoms, such as breathlessness. You may also want to make your own record of the drugs you're taking, dosage and any reactions to the medicines, keeping it in a way that makes sense to you.

Drug names

Drugs can have more than one name and this can confuse matters. There's the generic name, which is the chemical name for the drug, but each manufacturer will give their own name – a brand name – to their version of the drug. For instance, the generic name for gold injection is sodium aurothiomalate, but the company that produces this drug calls it Myocrisin.

Pregnancy

Talk to your doctor if you want to have children at some point as some of the drugs, such as the DMARDs, may cause problems to your developing baby. The risk of damage is greatest in the first three months of pregnancy. The normal rule is that you need to come off the drug for a time – usually three to six months before you start trying to conceive. Don't panic if you do accidentally become pregnant while on the DMARD as you're likely to have a healthy baby – the safety advice comes from studies on laboratory rats given very high doses of the drugs. This said, you need to seek advice from your doctor straight away about what to do regarding your drug treatments.

Sue was on penicillamine when she suddenly found out she was 14 weeks pregnant. 'I was very worried and went to see my doctor to discuss whether I should have a termination. But after talking through the risks I decided to continue with the pregnancy and I had a healthy baby girl.'

To help you cope with your symptoms during the time you're trying to become pregnant, you may be offered a low-dose steroid plus painkillers and a NSAID as these drugs are thought to be safe to take while trying for a baby. It's not always the case, but you may find it takes some time to conceive because the general effects of the disease may make you less fertile. If you can't cope without the DMARDs, you'll need to discuss what your options are with your doctor.

When you do become pregnant, you'll most likely find that your symptoms go, but they'll come back after the birth. Only a small number of women – perhaps 1 per cent – continue to have symptoms during pregnancy. Ideally, it's best not to take anything during pregnancy, but paracetamol is thought to be safe during this time and steroids may be prescribed, though other painkillers, NSAIDs and DMARDs shouldn't be taken.

Pat developed the disease after the birth of her first child, but found her symptoms went during her second pregnancy. 'I was so well I couldn't believe it and I didn't need any drugs. Everybody said I should be pregnant all the time. But my symptoms returned about 18 months after the birth of my second child.'

Breastfeeding

Many of the drugs can pass through breast milk to your baby, so, if you want to breastfeed, you need to check which drugs are safe to take. This issue is covered under each of the drugs, but the general advice is that low-dose steroids and paracetamol are thought to be safe. There may be problems with a few of the NSAIDs. Many of the DMARDs can be a problem, so you may not be able to breastfeed if you need to take one of these drugs.

The contraceptive pill

The combined pill and progestogen-only pill can be taken with most of the drugs and the pill's effectiveness shouldn't be affected. As with everything, though, double-check this with your doctor.

Male fertility

Many of the DMARDs can reduce sperm counts, though they don't affect sperm quality. If you're taking one of these drugs and it's taking a long time for your partner to become pregnant, it's important to have your sperm count checked. If it's low, talk to your doctor about your options. The solution may be to halve the drug dose or possibly stop taking the drug and, instead, take steroids, which shouldn't affect the sperm count. If the DMARD suits you, coming off it is not a decision to be taken lightly, as it's possible that when you go back on it, the drug may no longer work so well for you.

Depression

It's normal to feel low at times. The disease can affect all parts of your life and, if you can't do the things you want to, it's easy to become frustrated and depressed. Antidepressants can help you through difficult times so you may want to ask about which ones might be suitable for you. Be sure to check their side-effects. Antidepressants shouldn't interact with your other drugs but, again, double-check this.

Drugs and lovemaking

The drugs shouldn't affect your sex life, but if you've got any worries, talk to your doctor about them to discuss possible solutions. For instance, the disease can cause vaginal dryness if you develop Sjogren's syndrome, as can some of the antidepressants, so you may need to change antidepressants or use a vaginal lubricant.

Flare-ups

It's common for the disease to become more troublesome at times. You may feel very tired and washed out and experience more pain, stiffness and swelling than usual.

The drugs can be used in various ways to help you cope and this is discussed in more detail in the sections on the specific drugs, but it is important to note here that there are usually several main ways of dealing with flare-ups. It's a good idea to check these options out with your doctor in advance of having problems so that, if at all possible, you're prepared. For instance, if you take a NSAID, you may find you can settle a small flare-up by increasing the drug dose, though this clearly isn't an option if you're already taking the maximum daily dose. If you're on a DMARD, it may be possible to increase the dose, but it depends which drug you're on. You may even be able to increase the dose yourself, provided you've arranged this with your doctor in advance. Sometimes an intramuscular injection of a steroid drug is given to quickly settle a flare-up. If just one or two joints are affected, your doctor may give steroid injections into the joints. Your GP may prescribe low-dose steroid tablets if you can't get an appointment at the clinic for some time.

Children

Children may need to take a mixture of drugs – a painkiller, NSAID and a DMARD to bring the disease under control. Steroids can stunt growth, so check if any of the suitable steroid drugs are less likely to do this.

There have been concerns that the DMARDs can slightly affect a girl's fertility in the future, as the longer you're on one of these drugs the greater the chance it may affect your fertility. It's a grey area, but it's worth discussing the issue with your rheumatologist. (This is discussed in Chapter 4 with particular reference to methotrexate and cyclophosphamide.)

Vaccinations

If you're on a DMARD, you shouldn't be given a live vaccine. Alternative dead vaccines are normally available, but, if this isn't the case, you need to weigh up the pros and cons of a live vaccine against no vaccine with your doctor.

Holidays

It can be a worry if you think that your symptoms are going to worsen when you're away. Check with your doctor in advance if there is anything you can take with you to deal with potential problems. Some doctors, for instance, may give you a course of low-dose steroid tablets to take just in case of problems.

Hormone replacement therapy (HRT)

There shouldn't be any problem about taking HRT in combination with your rheumatoid arthritis drugs.

Bone health

The risk of osteoporosis – the bone-thinning disease – is greater if you're not that physically active and if you're taking steroids, as these drugs can cause bone thinning. HRT can prevent and treat bone loss and there are also non-hormonal drugs known as bisphosphonates that are used to treat osteoporosis. The various drugs should be safe to take with your other drugs, but double-check with your rheumatologist.

Try to look after your bones by keeping active and taking exercise. One way to reduce discomfort from exercise is to take a painkiller or NSAID tablet half an hour before exercising to minimize any discomfort (of course, you mustn't do this if it takes you over your daily maximum dose).

3

Painkillers and Non-steroidal Anti-inflammatory Drugs (NSAIDs)

Painkillers

What they do

Painkillers – 'analgesics' is the medical name for these drugs – curb pain, but they won't alter the disease process itself.

What's available?

Analgesics divide into two groups – the non-opioid ones and the opioid analgesics. Non-opioid drugs work by stopping the transmission of pain in the part of the body where you're experiencing pain. The opioids are related to opium, which is extracted from poppy seedheads. They work directly on the brain to alter your perception of pain. They're stronger than the non-opioids and are used for moderate to severe pain.

Options include paracetamol, which is a non-opioid drug available on and without prescription, and is good for mild to moderate pain. There are the codeine drugs, which are weak opioids, such as dihydrocodeine, also available on prescription. Next come the drugs that contain a mix of paracetamol and codeine, known as the combination drugs. These are available on prescription and include co-codamol (codeine and paracetamol) and co-dydramol (paracetamol and dihydrocodeine), co-proxamol (paracetamol and a mild opioid dextropropoxyphene). Solpadeine (paracetamol and codeine) is available without prescription and might be useful if you've run out of your normal combination tablets. Other options include Tramadol and Meptid, both opioid-like drugs, which are strong painkillers.

Note: Combination products that contain painkillers and NSAIDs are discussed later in this chapter under the heading How to take NSAIDs, as is aspirin.

What's best?

It's a case of finding which one suits you. Paracetamol on its own

21

is often not strong enough so many people find the combination products more useful. Some people take codeine regularly and add in paracetamol if the pain is bad, but it's important to know exactly what ingredients are in the painkillers you're taking so that you don't accidentally overdose. You might do this if, for instance, you take a combination product that contains paracetamol and then take additional paracetamol. See under Side-effects below.

How to take painkillers

You don't need to take painkillers regularly – just when you need them. Sometimes you may find you don't need to take them that much if you're going through a good phase, but you may need to take them regularly if you're in a lot of pain. As mentioned in the last chapter, it can be useful to top up with a painkiller about 30 minutes before you exercise to minimize potential discomfort.

Tip: In order to make sure you don't go over your daily dose, you could put your daily allowance (often eight tablets, but double-check this) in a bottle, then you can keep an accurate check on how many tablets you've taken.

Side-effects

Paracetamol doesn't irritate the stomach, nor should it cause constipation, though some people complain it does. It's seen as a safe drug, but it's important to follow safety instructions because paracetamol can cause liver and kidney damage, which can be fatal if you accidentally take an overdose. If you take paracetamol routinely and drink moderate amounts of alcohol regularly, your liver may be damaged, so you'll need to check with your doctor how much paracetamol you can have without causing problems.

Constipation can be a problem with the other painkillers. Try self-help measures, such as eating lots of prunes, plenty of fresh fruit and drinking plenty of fluids. If you need more help, ask about laxatives. If constipation is a real problem, ask about Tramadol. This also causes constipation, but less so than the opioid-based drugs, such as codeine, because Tramadol works in a different way. Drugs such as codeine can make you feel a bit sleepy and sometimes cause dizziness and a dry mouth. If they make you feel sick, try to take them with food. If this is a real problem, ask your doctor about anti-sickness tablets. There's also a risk that you could become dependent on the codeine drugs if you take them regularly, but this shouldn't be a problem with the combination products because they contain lower amounts of codeine.

Pregnancy

It's best to avoid taking any sort of drug when you're pregnant, though paracetamol is thought to be safe to take. Double-check what you can have with your doctor.

Breastfeeding

Paracetamol is considered safe to use when you're breastfeeding. With the other painkillers, double-check the position with your doctor. Often the situation is just not clear. For instance, no harmful effects have been reported for dihydrocodeine, but the drug companies that produce this drug say to use it while breastfeeding only if it's essential.

Painkillers and other medicines

Painkillers can usually be safely taken with the other drugs given for rheumatoid arthritis.

NSAIDs

These drugs are non-opioids. They're different from the group of drugs called painkillers and act by blocking the production of chemicals called prostaglandins, which cause inflammation. The drugs reduce swelling and stiffness in the joint lining and so also have a painkilling effect.

What's available?

There are quite a few NSAIDs and ones commonly prescribed include diclofenac, ibuprofen, naproxen and aceclofenac.

Note: Aspirin – one of the best-known painkillers – is a NSAID, but it's more likely to cause stomach problems than the other NSAIDs, particularly at the dose needed to produce an anti-inflammatory effect, so it isn't commonly used. If you've had no problems with aspirin, though, there's no reason to stop taking it – just be vigilant for possible side-effects. As both aspirin and other

NSAIDs can affect the kidneys, you shouldn't normally take the two together (but see the point about low-dose aspirin under the heading Who should avoid NSAIDs?).

There may be a choice of several different brands for each of the NSAIDs. Theoretically there should be no differences between the different versions of each drug but, in practice, you may find that one preparation suits you better than another, so it's worth asking whether or not there are any choices.

Mary had got on very well on one brand of naproxen, but then her prescription was changed. 'Within five days I developed a burning feeling inside my breast bone and I found out that I'd been put on another preparation of naproxen, so I was put back on the original brand and was fine.'

How to take NSAIDs

These drugs are usually taken in tablet form, though they're available sometimes as a suppository and can be given by injection. There are also NSAID creams and gels, but it's impractical to spread cream over large areas of your body on a regular basis and it's not clear that this is an effective way of getting the drug into your body.

Some people are very pleased with NSAIDs, but problems can occur at any time.

Sue took indomethacin for a couple of years, but had to stop when she developed dreadful headaches.

Jill found the drug very useful. 'I used an Indocid suppository each night for a long time. It was brilliant because I felt fine in the morning after a good night's sleep. But I can't use this any longer because the drug started to damage the lining of my back passage.'

There are also combination products that contain a painkiller and a NSAID, but these may not contain a sufficiently high dose of the NSAID to be effective for rheumatoid arthritis. However, Benorylate, which is a mix of aspirin and paracetamol, can work well.

Many people find they end up taking these drugs on a regular basis, though you may only need to take them occasionally if you're going through a good phase.

The drugs work quickly (within an hour) and last for different lengths of time depending on the drug and particular preparation. Naproxen, for example, lasts for around eight hours.

It's possible to take drugs that last longer in the body. Slow release, indicated by (SR) after the drug name, or retard, indicated by (R), are more slowly dissolved by the stomach and so can last for instance 12 or 24 hours. This can be very helpful if you get a lot of early morning stiffness.

It's important to know what your daily maximum dose is to get the best out of these drugs. For instance, if you do get a lot of problems first thing in the morning the following might be an option: take one 100 mg diclofenac retard tablet, which lasts for 24 hours, and in the morning top up with a 50 mg tablet, which takes you up to your 150 mg daily allowance for this drug. Double-check what you can do with your doctor.

Side-effects

NSAIDs can cause a number of side-effects, such as dizziness, as well as worsen asthma and heart problems. Do tell your doctor if you experience side-effects as there may be various solutions, such as changing to another drug or changing the dosage.

The drugs work by reducing the production of harmful prostaglandins, chemicals that cause inflammation in the body, but the problem is that they also reduce production of beneficial prostaglandins, which protect the stomach and kidneys. Stomach ulcers are an important side-effect.

Jane took Indocid occasionally for many years without any problems, but then became ill and was found to have a duodenal ulcer, so she had to stop taking the drug.

Jane's experience is fairly common – about 30 per cent of people on these drugs develop stomach problems. A stomach erosion, which is a break in the skin in the stomach lining, develops and this can become an ulcer, which is a more severe break in the skin that can penetrate blood vessels and cause bleeding.

Problems usually start within six months, but can, as Jane's story illustrates, occur at any time, even if you've been taking the drug for years. Warning symptoms include nausea, constant pain in the pit of the stomach and acid coming up into your mouth. If you lose blood, you may notice black, tarry stools or you may cough up blood and vomit may look dark and congealed. See your doctor straight away if any of these things happen.

Some doctors may want to do yearly kidney checks, whatever your age. However, if you're older, for instance over 60, your doctor may want to do regular six-monthly blood checks to see how your kidneys are working. The test looks at the levels of substances in the blood, such as urea and creatinine, that are normally eliminated from the body by healthy kidneys.

Your doctor needs to know if you suffer from asthma because NSAIDs can worsen asthma symptoms, though they can't cause asthma. You won't necessarily have any problems, but you'll be started on a lower than usual dose to see how you respond. If all is well, the dose will be increased. If you have problems, the solution may be to increase the dose of your asthma treatments. An alternative is to try ibuprofen at a low dose (400 mg three to four times a day) as this is likely to produce some benefit and reduce your chances of side-effects, such as bringing on your asthma symptoms. It's less powerful, but if you have the maximum 2.4-g daily dose, which is needed for a good, powerful effect, side-effects are more likely. An alternative might be the new COX-2 drugs mentioned below as these aren't supposed to worsen asthma.

NSAIDs can affect the colon so tell your doctor if you suffer from colitis, in which case you'll probably be started on a lower dose to see how you do. If problems occur, you may be put on low-dose ibuprofen.

Protecting your stomach

Take your NSAID dose with or after food. A drink and a couple of biscuits or slices of toast should be enough to line the stomach. Better still is to take the drug with or after a main meal.

If you're well into midlife (over 60), your doctor may prescribe drugs such as ranitidine (Zantac) or cimetidine (Tagamet), which reduce acid formation and so reduce the risk of an ulcer forming. Other types of drugs that reduce acid secretion include misoprostol and omeprazole. If the symptoms continue, a medicine called Gaviscon, which coats the stomach lining, may also be prescribed.

You could try combination products that contain a NSAID and antacid, such as Arthrotec (diclofenac and misoprostol).

If you're younger, your doctor is likely to wait and see if you develop problems. There are various things you can do to try to reduce acid production in your stomach, but it is impossible to guarantee that an ulcer won't develop:

- check the drug information as these drugs are usually best taken with or after a meal;
- stop smoking;
- reduce your alcohol intake;
- avoid spicy foods;
- eat a small rather than large meal at night.

If you still have problems, an antacid may be prescribed and Gaviscon.

It's also worth asking about enteric-coated preparations, which can help in a limited way by decreasing direct irritation of the stomach lining by the medication. This may slightly reduce the risk of nasty side-effects to the gut, but it's important to realize that side-effects will still occur once the drug has been broken down and absorbed into the circulation.

A suppository is another option, but, like the enteric-coated preparations, these can still cause side-effects, as in Jill's case.

If your symptoms persist, you'll need to have your stomach checked to make sure an ulcer isn't developing. This can be done by means of an endoscopy. You'll be given a mild sedative beforehand and then asked to swallow a slim, flexible tube that enables the lining of the oesophagus (known commonly as the gullet), the stomach and the duodenum to be seen. An alternative is a barium meal. This involves swallowing a bland white liquid. An X-ray is then taken and any ulcers will show up as craters.

These tests may show that your symptoms are due, not to an ulcer, but to acid reflux. This is when digestive juices containing acid rise back up into the gullet. If this happens a lot, the gullet can become inflamed. Reflux occurs when the valve at the entrance to the stomach becomes weak. Smoking, drinking coffee and eating fats can temporarily weaken the valve and, if you do any of these things a lot, can result in acid reflux, commonly called heartburn. The valve can also become weakened if you're overweight.

If you have got acid reflux, you'll be put on an acid-blocking drug. If you're already on one, the dose may be increased or you may be put on another antacid.

If an ulcer is developing, you will have to stop taking any NSAIDs.

Note: There are two new NSAIDs – celecoxib and rofecoxib, known as COX-2-specific inhibitors. These are discussed in more detail in Chapter 6. However, drugs such as meloxicam (Mobic) have been around for several years and are the first of this class of drugs, which aim to shut off the harmful prostaglandins without stopping production of the beneficial prostaglandins. It's worth talking to your doctor about drugs such as Mobic, though you may still have problems with these drugs.

NSAIDs and other medicines

These drugs can often be taken with many other drugs, but there are interactions with certain other ones. For example, drugs called ACE inhibitors, which lower blood pressure, won't work so well if you also take NSAIDs. So it's important to double-check what the position is for any other prescription drugs, as well as over-the-counter medicines.

NSAIDs are usually safe to take with painkillers and with DMARDs, and they won't affect the efficacy of the contraceptive pill. They can also be taken with steroids, but, as steroids can also affect your stomach, it may be a good idea to take an antacid if you're taking a steroid as well as a NSAID – check this with your doctor. Note that it's best not to take aspirin as this is also a NSAID with the same side-effects, but there are exceptions – see the comment on low-dose aspirin under the next heading.

You shouldn't normally take a NSAID if you take the blood-thinning drug warfarin, because NSAIDs can cause stomach erosions and if your blood is thinner, you'll bleed more easily.

Who should avoid NSAIDs?

These drugs are not advisable if you've got a history of ulcers, severe asthma, colitis, kidney failure or you're taking warfarin.

If you're taking low-dose aspirin (150 mg) each day – to protect against stroke or heart problems, for example – you may be able to take a NSAID, but you need to check whether you can with your doctor as aspirin also affects the stomach.

Pregnancy

Stop taking the drug as soon as you know you're pregnant as the drug can affect placental blood flow to the baby.

Breastfeeding

Always double-check what the latest advice is for the drug you're taking, though there may be no clear evidence on this point.

Some of the drugs, such as diclofenac and ibuprofen, are considered safe. However, traces of diclofenac do pass through breast milk, so it may not be as safe as ibuprofen which doesn't.

Indomethacin should be avoided or used with caution as small amounts are excreted in breast milk. These amounts are probably too small to be harmful, but there is one reported case of it causing convulsions in a breastfed baby.

It's unknown whether or not meloxicam passes into breast milk, so the advice is to avoid it.

There's conflicting advice about naproxen, so it's best to avoid it, and the same is true for nabumetone.

Flare-ups

Possible options include increasing the drug dosage if there's leeway – that is, you've not reached your maximum daily dose – but you can't do this if you're already taking the maximum amount.

Alcohol

Alcohol in moderation is fine, but it can irritate the stomach, so be careful not to overdo it.

4

Disease-modifying Anti-rheumatic Drugs (DMARDs)

There are various types of drugs in this group, but they all share one action: they have some effect on the underlying disease process. They don't cure the disease but control it and, as mentioned in Chapter 2, aren't painkillers but can reduce pain by halting the underlying disease process.

They're powerful drugs that can have potentially serious side-effects, and many affect how well your immune system works. It's difficult to know in advance whether a drug will work for you because something that works well for someone else may not work for you and vice versa or it may work but you suffer bad side-effects.

DMARDs are extremely important drugs because they can be very effective at slowing down the disease process, which means you're less likely to need joint surgery or tendon repair at some later date. Many people with rheumatoid arthritis will need to take these drugs. Indeed, it's estimated that 98 per cent of 45-year-olds with the disease will need them.

Note that these drugs do take time to work and you'll have to be carefully monitored when you're on them because of their possible side-effects. It's a case of weighing up the advantages and disadvantages of the various drugs with your doctor.

Early treatment

As explained in Chapter 2, these drugs used to be reserved for use later on in the disease, but now that it's known that joint damage occurs early in the disease your doctor is likely to want you to try one of these drugs as soon as you've been diagnosed.

Jill wishes she had been put on the drugs when she was first diagnosed as having the disease over 30 years ago. 'For the first four years my GP kept saying the disease would burn out and he just gave me a few aspirin to take. Then I was referred to a rheumatologist who was reluctant to put me on what he described as the heavy drugs unless I really needed them.

Fifteen years ago when my symptoms got really bad I was put on gold and it's worked very well for me ever since. If they'd put me on this treatment much earlier on my joints probably wouldn't have been so badly affected.'

Despite this, these are powerful drugs and you should only be put on them if it's certain that you do have rheumatoid arthritis. This fact highlights the need for an accurate diagnosis, as discussed in Chapter 1.

When might these drugs be suggested?

Practice tends to vary a bit between rheumatologists, but there are various situations in which it's likely your specialist will recommend these drugs, such as the following.

- There are no hard-and-fast rules, but it's well known that the disease is usually more problematic if it starts when you're in midlife, so many people in this group will need these drugs.
- If you have a raised ESR (erythrocyte sedimentation rate) – a sign that there is inflammation – a lot of early morning stiffness and the specialist finds evidence of swelling in at least one joint.
- There's evidence of joint inflammation – that is, puffy joints in the pattern characteristic of rheumatoid arthritis, described under the heading Symptoms in Chapter 1.
- Erosions show up on your X-ray, even though your symptoms may be well under control and the rheumatologist finds no obvious swelling.
- If you develop vasculitis or have a flare-up in the disease, even if it's been well controlled before without DMARDs.
- If you've developed rheumatoid nodules and have a very high rheumatoid factor level as well as swollen joints.

However, your doctor is likely to adopt a 'wait and see' policy if you've got painful joints but the rheumatologist can't find any evidence of inflammation on examination of your joints and your X-rays are normal.

The types of drugs available

The immunosuppressant drugs are methotrexate, azathioprine, cyclosporin, cyclophosphamide, chlorambucil, leflunomide (which became available in 1999); the antimalarial drug hydroxychloroquine; gold; sulphasalazine; penicillamine; the new biological

31

drugs infliximab (Remicade) and etanercept (Enbrel), which were licensed early in 2000, and are discussed in Chapter 6.

How long do you need to stay on these drugs?

The drugs don't cure the disease, so, even if one works for you and you have no side-effects, you still need to take it. There's some evidence that people who stop taking these drugs are nearly twice as likely to have a flare-up within a year compared to people who continue the treatment. However, you need to come off the drug if it stops working or causes nasty side-effects. If this happens, your doctor will want to try you on another one of these drugs.

The choice of drugs

You may think from looking at the list of drugs that you've got a big choice, but this isn't really so. It's quite common for a DMARD to work for only three to four years and then you'll need to change to another one – this happens to around 80 per cent of people – but you may find the next drug doesn't work for you or you suffer bad side-effects. So, it's important to stay on the drug for as long as it works for you. If you have a break from the drug and then go back on it you may find it no longer works for you, as Helen's story illustrates.

'I started on gold injections ten years ago. The gold worked very well for me for about five years, so the doctors took me off gold because they thought the disease was under control. But three months afterwards my fingers became swollen and I felt really poorly and had all sorts of skin problems. I was put back on the gold, but it didn't work for me and I had awful side-effects – my left wrist was like a piece of raw meat. Since then I've tried other drugs but they haven't worked.'

This isn't always the case, however, and women who need to come off these drugs because they're pregnant often find they can have a break and go back on the drug again without any problems.

Let us now look at the main DMARDs in more detail.

Methotrexate (immunosuppressant)

Don't be alarmed if you've heard that this is a cancer drug. It's used to treat some types of cancer, but, for the last ten years or so, it's also been used at much lower doses to treat rheumatoid arthritis. At the moment, it's probably one of the drugs of first choice, alongside sulphasalazine, which doctors also use to control rheumatoid arthritis.

How it works

It's not clear exactly how the drug works, but it seems to reduce the amount of new joint lining manufactured, which, in turn, means that fewer inflammatory agents called cytokines are produced. It also affects the immune system. The end result is that it reduces the development of erosions on the bones of the joints.

When it's used

It's a powerful prescription-only drug used for all age groups, particularly if there's active disease. This last point means it's often used for children as they tend to have more active disease.

What to expect

It can start to work as quickly as three weeks after you start to take it, but, then again, you may not feel any benefit for three months.

The starting dose is often 7.5 mg, normally taken as three 2.5-mg tablets once a week, with the dose increasing to around 15 mg weekly if all is well. It can even go up to 25 mg weekly, though this is rare.

A divided dose is sometimes advised if your symptoms are very bad by the time you're about to take your next weekly dose. Then, the dose is split into two, one half being taken at the beginning of the week and the remainder some time later that week. This can provide better symptom relief. It's worth discussing this option with your doctor if you find that taking the tablets in one go doesn't quite tide you over the seven days. Very rarely, methotrexate may be taken daily. It's not a painkiller, so you need to keep taking your other drugs as these provide relief from symptoms.

Side-effects

These include an upset stomach, liver damage, mouth ulcers, thinning hair, thickening of lung tissue, though this isn't common, possibly an itchy rash, a less effective immune system and bruising easily. It's not known whether there are any cancer risks linked to this drug at the moment.

Because the drug is broken down by the liver, it's not likely to be suitable for someone who is a heavy drinker (the liver would then become overloaded) or has liver disease. Before you go on the drug, various tests are done to check the state of your liver.

If you have lung problems, you may be able to take the drug, but you'll need extra lung tests, such as chest X-rays. The rheumatologist may then want to refer you to a chest physician if there are concerns about the test results.

Nausea is a common side-effect, but there are various things you can do to minimize this, so discuss these with your doctor. For instance, take your dose after food or take an anti-sickness tablet in the 24-hour period in which you take your methotrexate dose. Another option is to have a divided dose, as mentioned above. If you suffer a lot of sickness and none of these suggestions, or others that your doctor might have, help, then ask about intramuscular injections. These are given in hospital and may be the answer, though injections are not always practical because they involve frequent visits to hospital and are more expensive so they're not often offered. Another possible solution is to reduce the methotrexate dose and to add in another DMARD.

You may start to get mouth ulcers and thinner hair because the drug depletes levels of folic acid in the body. In order to reduce these side-effects, most doctors nowadays advise you to take folic acid supplements as soon as you start on methotrexate. Practice varies, but, for instance, if you're on a 10-mg dose, you may be advised to take a 5-mg folic acid supplement 48 hours before you take the methotrexate or to take a folic acid tablet daily except on the day you take the methotrexate.

About one in ten people develop methotrexate nodules. These are lumpy bits under the skin that often develop around pressure points, such as the elbows and backs of the heels. The nodules can develop rapidly in the first months of starting on the drug. Treatment options include taking hydroxychloroquine with the methotrexate, as there's some evidence that this DMARD can reduce or prevent the formation of the nodules, or else reducing the methotrexate dose. The nodules can be removed surgically, though they often regrow.

Methotrexate and other medicines

It can be co-prescribed with other DMARDs, but not with penicillamine.

There's also a theoretical concern that the drug can interact with NSAIDs, making the methotrexate more potent – that is, the NSAID displaces the methotrexate from proteins, which frees up the methotrexate in the circulation, making it more powerful. However, in practice, most rheumatologists do prescribe the two types of drugs together and it's very rare for there to be any problems.

The drug doesn't interact with the contraceptive pill.

Monitoring

A full blood count and liver function test will be done before you go on the drug. If there are concerns about your liver and it's important for you to go on this drug, a tissue sample called a liver biopsy is taken under local anaesthetic to find out more about the state of your liver.

In some clinics, your lungs will be checked by means of a chest X-ray and lung function tests, but this doesn't always happen if you don't already have chest problems.

If all is well, you'll have regular checks once you start taking the drug, including a full blood count and liver tests to see how your liver is coping with the drug. If liver enzymes rise by more than three times the pre-treatment level, your doctor may reduce the drug dosage or you may have to stop taking the drug. These tests may be done fortnightly for the first six weeks, then on a monthly basis if all is well. ESR levels are also likely to be checked at various points to measure disease activity.

Apart from the monitoring tests, let your doctor know if you develop any problems. For instance, about one in twenty people develop breathlessness because the drug can thicken lung tissue. If this happens, contact the clinic so that tests can be done to check what's happening to your lungs.

Your immune system may not be working so well because of the drug, so try to avoid contact with people who have infections. If you start to succumb to more infections and fevers than you used to, contact the clinic to get your white count checked. If there is a problem, your drug dosage may be reduced, but, if this doesn't help, you may need to come off the drug. Also, if you've not had chickenpox before, try to avoid anyone who has this or shingles. If you do come into contact with someone who has either of these, let your doctor know in case you need special treatment.

Pregnancy

You shouldn't become pregnant while taking methotrexate. The normal advice if you want to start a family is to stop taking the drug and have a break of six months, during which time you use contraception, before trying for a baby. If you do become pregnant while taking the drug, don't panic – it's unlikely that abnormalities will have occurred in your developing baby because of the low doses used to treat rheumatoid arthritis. Don't take your next dose if it's due, and seek advice from your clinic or GP about what you should do, within 24 hours if possible.

Breastfeeding

You shouldn't breastfeed your baby if you're taking this drug because it is excreted in small amounts in breast milk and may build up in your baby.

Fertility

Methotrexate can reduce sperm count in men, so you may need to stop taking the drug if you've been trying for a while and your partner is still not pregnant.

There's no hard evidence for this, but some doctors worry that the drug may also slightly affect female fertility, so, if you want to have children in the next year or so and don't have active disease, your doctor may prescribe sulphasalazine instead, as this isn't thought to affect fertility.

However, your doctor will want you to take methotrexate if you've got active disease. If you need to take the drug but want to protect your fertility, talk to your doctor about whether going on the contraceptive pill would help. The logic behind this is that the eggs in your ovaries are less exposed to the drug because you don't ovulate. However, there's little research about the usefulness of doing this for methotrexate, although some doctors suggest this strategy for the drug cyclophosphamide, discussed later in this chapter.

If you forget to take your tablets

It's a good idea to ask about this in advance so that you know what to do if it happens. The usual advice is that you can take your dose up to two days later and then just go back to your normal regime.

Flare-ups

Check in advance what to do if your symptoms flare up so that, if possible, you're prepared for this. Options may include:

- temporarily increasing the dose by adding in an extra 2.5-mg methotrexate tablet;
- increasing the NSAID dose if there's scope to – that is, you're not already on the maximum dose;
- having a steroid injection or taking a short course of low-dose steroid tablets.

Once the flare-up has settled down, you simply go back to your normal regime. If you keep getting flare-ups, you may need to stay on a higher methotrexate dose or, in addition to the methotrexate, be given another DMARD to help control the disease, or else come off methotrexate.

If you have mouth ulcers and they get worse, you may need more folic acid or take a lower methotrexate dose.

If you stop taking the drug

No harm will come to you if you stop taking the drug, though your symptoms are likely to worsen once you're off it. If you don't want to stay on the drug, it's best to talk to your doctor about what other options there are rather than just stop taking it.

Vaccinations

Dead ones are best and live vaccines should be avoided if possible, as discussed in Chapter 2.

Alcohol

Go easy on alcohol because it puts pressure on the liver, as does the drug. Discuss what you can safely drink with your doctor.

Sulphasalazine

This is the drug of first or second choice. It has been used for about the last 15 years to treat the disease, but it's not clear how it works, even though it was developed specifically as an anti-rheumatic drug, unlike many of the other DMARDs.

The brand prescribed is Salazopyrin EN which is enteric coated – that is, it has been specially coated to reduce stomach problems. As mentioned earlier under the heading Fertility in the section on methotrexate, there's no firm evidence, but some doctors are concerned that methotrexate may reduce future female fertility. That is, you may find it more difficult to conceive once you have been on and then stop taking the drug and try for a baby. Sulphasalazine shouldn't affect your future fertility, so it may be prescribed in preference to methotrexate for those wanting to start a family in the future or young girls with moderately active disease (but methotrexate is usually the drug of first choice if there's active disease).

What to expect

A typical starting dose is 1 gram, taken as two 500-mg tablets daily for a fortnight to a month. If you're well on this, the dose is usually doubled to 1 gram in the morning and 1 gram in the evening.

It can take up to three months for it to start to work and you may feel a bit nauseous for a few weeks, though this normally settles down, so keep taking it. Try it with food or after food to minimize nausea symptoms or talk to your doctor about taking a slightly lower dose and spreading it over the day – for example, three 500-mg tablets, taking one at breakfast, one at lunch and one in the evening. Remember that it's not a painkiller so you need to keep taking your other drugs that provide symptom relief.

Side-effects

It's a relatively safe drug that most people can take and serious side-effects are uncommon. Even so, it's not for everyone.

Pat was on it for a year. 'It helped and my joints were better but my mouth became ulcerated and I felt irritable and a bit run down. In the end I said I couldn't take it any more.'

As noted earlier, sulphasalazine can cause stomach problems, also skin rashes, diarrhoea and may affect your platelet count so that you bruise more easily.

It may reduce your blood count and make you more susceptible to infections, so, if you keep getting lots of infections, sore throats or fevers or you're taking longer to recover from illnesses, you'll need your white blood count checked. If there's a problem, the drug dose may be halved or you may need to come off the drug altogether. There aren't any cancer risks with this drug.

The drug can make your urine and tears go an orange colour, though this doesn't happen to everyone. If you wear soft contact lenses, it's possible these may become slightly orange, but it's very unlikely and is not harmful.

If you develop an itchy, eczema-like rash, see your doctor or GP in the first instance for advice about what to do. If it's very bad, you may not be able to keep taking this drug.

Sulphasalazine and other medicines

There aren't any significant problems with other drugs and it doesn't interact with the contraceptive pill. However, always double-check whether or not any new medicine you're about to take interacts with sulphasalazine.

Monitoring

A full blood count and liver function test are done before you start on the drug and then they are repeated at regular intervals once you're taking it. A typical regime might be fortnightly tests for the first six weeks and then at three-monthly intervals, assuming all is well.

ESR levels may be measured at quarterly intervals to check how active the disease is and see how well the drug is working.

The liver breaks down the drug and so if liver enzymes become three times higher than the pre-treatment level, the dose will be reduced or you may need to come off it.

Pregnancy

You shouldn't get pregnant while taking this drug. The usual advice is to stop taking it three months before you want to try for a baby and use contraception in the interval as it could affect the developing baby. If you do accidentally become pregnant while you're taking the drug, there's no need to panic, but contact your clinic for advice straight away.

Breastfeeding

Talk to your doctor about whether or not it's safe to breastfeed while taking this drug as it's excreted in breast milk.

Fertility

It can reduce the sperm count, though this should recover after stopping sulphasalazine, but shouldn't affect female fertility, after coming off the drug.

If you forget to take your tablets

Check in advance with your clinic what you should do if this happens. It is not something to get anxious about. The usual advice if you forget to take your daily tablets is just to carry on as normal the next day, not to double up the dose. If you realize that you forgot to take your morning dose when you're about to take the evening dose, just take the evening tablets. However, if you remember at midday that you've forgotten the morning dose, take the tablets then and, later on, take the evening tablets as usual.

Flare-ups

If you keep getting flare-ups, you may be put on the maximum daily dose, which is 3 grams. This extra amount will take time to work, so you may be given a steroid injection or low-dose steroid tablets to tide you over until the higher dose starts to work. Another option is to increase your NSAID dose if there's scope – that is, if you're not already taking the maximum amount.

Vaccinations

Avoid live vaccines, opting for dead ones if possible.

Alcohol

Sulphasalazine is broken down by the liver, so you do need to be careful about how much alcohol you drink. Check with your doctor what you can safely drink.

Leflunomide (immunosuppressant)

This drug (Arava) became available in the autumn of 1999 and is the first new DMARD to be introduced in the UK for more than ten years. It's powerful, with supposedly fewer side-effects than some of the other DMARDs. Studies suggest that it could be the drug of third choice or even move higher up the list, and one study suggested it was as good as methotrexate. However, its real value and side-effects will only become apparent once it's been used for some time by lots of people in the general community.

Note: At the moment, it's licensed only for people aged 18 and over.

Sue has been on leflunomide for several months. She developed the disease nine years ago and has been on various drugs, including methotrexate, but developed a dreadful itchy rash all over her legs when she was on this. She went on to Arava because other drugs weren't working for her. She also takes a low-dose steroid tablet each day. 'So far Arava has been wonderful and I can do a lot more things now. I don't have stiffness in the mornings and I can have a shower without wondering whether I can stand long enough to have one. I haven't had any side-effects, the pain has pretty much gone and I feel good. I just take the occasional painkiller whereas I took them all the time before.'

How it works

It reduces the ability of lymphocytes (white blood cells, which are part of the immune system) to produce pain, inflammation and joint damage.

What to expect

The initial dose is what's known as a loading dose – that is, a higher dose is given to boost the effect of the drug as a lower dose might take longer to have an effect. Thus, 100 mg a day is taken for the first three days and this is reduced to a 10–20-mg tablet taken once a day. There's no step-up dose and the drug can start to work as early as four weeks after starting to take it. Remember that it's not a painkiller, so you need to keep taking your other drugs that provide symptom relief.

Side-effects

Leflunomide is reported to have fewer side-effects than some of the other DMARDs. The commonest are digestive ones, so it may be best to take it with food to prevent nausea or last thing at night with an anti-sickness pill. Discuss this with your doctor if you're having problems.

Other side-effects include diarrhoea, which can be a problem, particularly with the higher-loading dose. If this happens to you, you could try going down to the normal maintenance dose – that is,

20 mg rather than staying on the 100-mg daily dose – for three days. However, this means the drug will take longer to work – perhaps not having an effect for two months. Alternatively, you could ask your doctor for anti-diarrhoea treatments while you're on the loading dose.

You may also find you suffer from abdominal pain, a skin rash (if it's very uncomfortable, this may mean you can't keep taking the drug), hypertension (raised blood pressure), weight loss, temporary hair loss while on the drug, raised levels of liver enzymes (in which case the dose may be reduced to 10 mg daily), and allergic reactions. The drug can also affect your bone marrow, so you may get a low white blood count. Again, if you're on a higher (20-mg) dose, this may be reduced to 10 mg.

If you've not had chickenpox before, try to avoid contact with anyone who has it or shingles. If you do come into contact with someone who has either of these, let your doctor know in case you need special treatment.

It's not known at the moment whether or not there are any risks of cancer with leflunomide.

It's not advisable for someone who has got marked liver disease or severe kidney disease to take this drug.

Leflunomide and other medicines

Check with your doctor. Leflunomide is metabolized by the liver and it also suppresses bone marrow so taking any other drugs that do either of these things as well as leflunomide might be problematical.

Leflunomide should not be co-prescribed with methotrexate nor with sulphasalazine, but it's not known yet whether it can also be taken with the new biological drugs discussed in Chapter 6. It shouldn't affect the contraceptive pill.

Monitoring

You need to have your blood pressure measured, a full blood count done and your liver enzyme levels checked before going on the drug. Once you're on the drug, it's currently recommended that your blood pressure should continue to be checked from time to time (every month or so), though how often will depend on whether or not you have a history of blood pressure problems. Equally, full blood count tests should be done every two weeks for the first six months of treatment and then every eight weeks from then on. Also, you will need to have the liver function tests repeated probably every month for the first six months and then every eight weeks.

Pregnancy

The drug can stay in your body for up to two years so men and women wanting to start a family need to stop taking leflunomide (Arava) and take cholestyramine or activated charcoal (though you need to check whether or not these can affect any other drugs you're taking) for 11 days as a way of getting the drug out of your body quickly. The most recent advice is that, after this time, men can try for a baby straight away. Women are advised to wait for one full menstrual cycle before trying to conceive, but it may be safer to allow at least three months before trying as this is a new drug and it's not known exactly how it'll affect the developing baby. Double-check with your doctor on this and ask if you can have a blood test to check whether or not the drug is still in your body. If you do accidentally become pregnant while still taking the drug, don't take the next dose and speak to your doctor or clinic about your situation within 24 hours, if possible.

Breastfeeding

Don't breastfeed while taking this drug.

Fertility

It's not known at the moment whether or not this drug might reduce the sperm count in men. It's unlikely to affect female fertility.

If you forget to take your tablets

Don't worry – just take your normal dose the next day. Don't double up to compensate for the dose you missed the previous day.

Flare-ups

Options include increasing the dose of your NSAID or painkillers or else being given steroid treatment.

Vaccinations

The advice is the same as for the other DMARDs – avoid live vaccines if at all possible.

43

Alcohol

As this drug is broken down by the liver, you need to be careful about how much alcohol you can have. Check with your doctor how much you can safely drink.

Gold

This has been used for over 60 years to treat rheumatoid arthritis. It's a powerful drug that comes high up the list of drug treatments of choice, though it's not exactly clear how it works and it has potentially serious side-effects.

It can work as well as methotrexate and sulphasalazine, but these other drugs are easier to administer because they're usually taken in tablet form whereas gold is usually given by injection in hospital.

If you want to try the drug because, for instance, your mother found it worked for her, then ask your doctor if you can do so. It's used for people of all ages. Sometimes it helps and other times it doesn't.

Pat had a severe reaction and needed to be hospitalized. 'I got up to a 50-mg dose and then the trouble started and I got an awful itchy rash all over my body. I struggled with this for about six weeks and finally saw my rheumatologist who took one look at me and put me in hospital. I was put on steroid tablets to calm everything down.'

Jill, 64, started on gold 15 years ago. 'I was in so much pain that I was happy to try the gold. I remember starting on it and thinking after six weeks that it wasn't going to work, but, after three months on gold, the pain started to go and the swelling went down. It's worked wonders for me and I've never had any side-effects with it and I'll stay on it as long as it works.'

Mary was reluctant to try gold because of worries about side-effects, but eventually she tried it. 'It took about five months to see any improvement, but I got a lot better and was in less pain and looked younger and better and I had no side-effects. But after a couple of years my symptoms got worse and I was put on fortnightly gold treatment, but in the end gold stopped working for me.'

Sue got some relief from gold for four months, but then suddenly seized up with pain and had to be taken to hospital because she couldn't move.

What to expect

Gold is usually given by injection and the preparation is called sodium aurothiomalate (Myocrisin). It does come in tablet form – auranofin – but tablets can cause digestive upsets, so they're not usually prescribed. Also, some specialists think that the tablets are less powerful than the injections.

It may take three months or longer before you notice any benefit. It's not a painkiller, so you need to keep taking your other drugs that provide symptom relief.

Side-effects

These include rashes, which must always be reported to your doctor as they can be a sign of a serious reaction; also, protein in the urine and abnormal blood counts. A rare problem is colitis.

Gold isn't linked to an increased risk of any cancers.

If the gold isn't quite suppressing your symptoms, say so, as the injection may be given at three-weekly intervals, provided your body is coping with the drug well.

If you're doing well on gold but your blood count is a bit low, injections may be given at five-weekly intervals.

If you get nasty mouth ulcers as a side-effect, again the solution may be to have five-weekly injections.

Bruising easily can be a side-effect if the drug has affected your platelet count. Ask your doctor what can be done about this.

Mention if you're getting more breathless. There are various reasons for this. Gold can lead to thickening of the tissue inside the lung, though this is pretty rare, or kidney problems, which are more common, so it is important to be watchful.

Gold and other medicines

It's generally safe with other drugs and doesn't affect the contraceptive pill, but always double-check any possible drug interactions with your doctor and pharmacist.

Monitoring

The drug is given under careful scrutiny in case you develop serious problems. Twenty-four hours before you start to take the drug you'll have a full blood count. Your urine will be carefully checked, too, because gold is broken down by the kidneys and one of its side-effects is excessive protein leaking into the urine – a sign that the kidneys aren't working well. Some specialists also do a blood test to check for substances such as serum creatinine, which is normally eliminated from the body by healthy kidneys. If there are any queries about your results, more tests will be done. If there are any problems, you may not be able to take gold. If kidney problems develop once you're on gold, the dose may be halved or you may have to come off the drug.

If your initial tests are clear, then you'll have a 10-mg test dose – a painless injection into the buttock to see how you react to this. If you have no reactions, you'll be given a higher 50-mg dose weekly for around 20 weeks until you've had 1,000 mg (1 gram) of gold. If the gold is helping, you'll normally have a 50-mg (maintenance dose) monthly injection. However, treatment should be stopped if the gold hasn't helped you by this point.

Monitoring tests are carried out prior to the injection at weekly, or possibly fortnightly, intervals and then monthly once your injections are monthly. They are very important, so make sure you have your checks. You'll probably be given a monitoring book that will record how much gold you've received in total. There's no maximum limit and if the drug works you can stay on it indefinitely.

Early warning signs of intolerance of the drug include mouth ulcers, which can be quite bad, and a nasty rash (see under Side-effects, above). It is important to let your doctor know straight away if you develop any symptoms.

Pregnancy

You shouldn't become pregnant while you are being treated with gold. It's also best to come off the drug and have a three-month gap before trying for a baby. If you do become pregnant while on gold, though, stay calm and see your doctor as soon as possible.

Breastfeeding

It's best to play safe and not breastfeed when you're receiving gold treatment.

Fertility

As far as is known, it's not thought to affect male or female fertility in any way.

Flare-ups

If there's scope – that is, you're not already being given the maximum dose – your doctor is likely to try increasing the dose of your painkiller or NSAID. If this doesn't help or isn't possible, your doctor may prescribe low-dose steroid tablets, a steroid injection or joint injections if only one or two joints are affected.

If you keep having flare-ups, you may need to change to a different DMARD as you can't have more than the 50-mg dose and it's very unusual to have fortnightly injections.

Another option may be that your doctor suggests you take hydroxychloroquine with the gold.

Vaccinations

Avoid live vaccines and opt for dead ones instead if possible.

Alcohol

There shouldn't be a problem as gold is metabolized by the kidneys.

Hydroxychloroquine (an anti-malarial drug)

Anti-malarial drugs were found to be useful for treating rheumatoid arthritis by accident.

The most commonly prescribed one is hydroxychloroquine (Plaquenil). It's not a powerful drug, but it's good for mild rheumatoid arthritis and is used for all age groups. However, it's likely your doctor will want to prescribe a stronger DMARD if you're young.

It's usually prescribed with another DMARD drug in the following situations:

- if the other drug isn't effective enough on its own and increasing the dosage might increase its side-effects, hydroxychloroquine might be used as a 'helper' to boost the effectiveness of the other drug;

- it may be prescribed with methotrexate to reduce or prevent the formation of methotrexate nodules.

What to expect

It's taken by tablet, often a 200-mg tablet daily. The drug doesn't start to have any effect until three months or so after you start taking it. It's not a painkiller, so continue to take your other drugs that provide symptom relief.

Side-effects

Hydroxychloroquine is seen as a relatively safe drug. Side-effects may include stomach upsets, you may feel a bit nauseous for a couple of hours after taking the drug and it can leave a bitter taste in the mouth. So swallow the tablet whole with water around a mealtime.

Other side-effects include headaches and bruising more easily. The drug can also affect the bone marrow, though this is rare.

The main problem is that it can affect your skin. It's possible for over-pigmentation of the skin to develop so, for instance, you get brown blotches if you have white skin or black blotches if you have brown or black skin. Also, you may get under-pigmentation of the skin, which can cause pale blotches to appear in coloured skin. The problem doesn't just happen on skin exposed to the sun – it can also affect the tongue and tissue around the gums. Try to protect against this by covering up in the sunshine, using sun block and wear a wide-brimmed hat to protect your face. If skin problems start to develop, contact your GP or rheumatology clinic because they may be irreversible so it may not be a good idea to stay on the drug.

Hydroxychloroquine can also affect the retinas, which are at the back of the eye, and may worsen the symptoms of the skin disease psoriasis.

The drug may not be suitable for you if you've got heart problems.

It's not linked to any cancers.

Hydroxychloroquine and other medicines

It can be taken with many other drugs, including the DMARDs and it doesn't affect the contraceptive pill. However, if you take drugs for a muscle weakness disorder called myasthenia gravis, you may not be able to take hydroxychloroquine as the various drugs used to treat it interact with hydroxychloroquine and your muscle weakness symptoms could worsen.

Indigestion remedies – antacids – can reduce absorption of the drug. They can also make it more powerful because the antacids and the anti-malarial drug are both broken down by the liver, so double-check what you should do with your doctor or a pharmacist. The advice may be to have a four-hour gap between taking the antacid and the hydroxychloroquine. The drug can also make the heart drug digoxin more powerful, so tell your doctor if you're on this.

Monitoring

There aren't strong guidelines about what tests should be done if you're on this drug. Eye examinations by an ophthalmologist (a doctor who specializes in eye problems) used to be advised, but now these checks are not considered necessary if you take one tablet a day, which is what most people take. However, some rheumatologists may still advise you to have your eyes checked none the less.

Regardless of dose, however, you should have your eyes checked if you have eye problems before going on the drug or if you develop blurred vision or problems while taking it. If, for some reason, you're taking two tablets a day, it's likely your rheumatologist will recommend you have your eyes checked regularly by an ophthalmologist.

If you don't fall into any of these categories and you don't have any obvious problems on the drug, it's probably still a good idea to have your eyes checked once a year as a precaution, and your optician should be able to do this – make sure they know you're taking this drug.

Hydroxychloroquine isn't a powerful drug so it doesn't affect the blood count very often. However, as a precaution, your doctor may do six-monthly full blood counts as the drug can reduce the bone marrow's ability to make new cells.

Pregnancy

Don't become pregnant if you can help it while on this drug. Come off it and have a three- to six-month gap before you try for a family.

Breastfeeding

It's best not to because the drug is excreted in small amounts of breast milk.

Fertility

It doesn't appear to affect male or female fertility.

If you forget to take your tablets

Don't double up the next day's dose if you forget to take one day's daily dose. There aren't any sudden withdrawal symptoms or side-effects if you suddenly stop taking this drug – for example, if you forget to take it on a week's holiday – because the effects of the drug take quite a long time to wear off.

Flare-ups

Increase the dose of your NSAID if there's scope to do so. There's no evidence that increasing the hydroxychloroquine dose to two tablets a day is of benefit, but discuss the options with your doctor.

Vaccinations

Avoid live vaccines, opting for dead ones if possible.

Alcohol

Check what you can safely drink with your doctor, though there shouldn't be a particular problem.

Azathioprine (immunosuppressant)

Azathioprine (Imuran) inhibits the action of lymphocytes – those white cells that are part of the immune system and can cause inflammation.

It's a weaker drug, like hydroxychloroquine, so it's not usually the drug of first choice, coming further down the list. It's often used as a helper – that is, to boost the effectiveness of another DMARD, though it may be used on its own if none of the other drugs works for you. It may also be prescribed together with steroids if you develop vasculitis (inflammation of the blood vessels) or be used to suppress vasculitis while you come off steroids.

What to expect

It's taken as a tablet and the dose given relates to your weight, so you'll be weighed before you start on the drug. A usual starting dose is 2.5 mg per kilogram (approximately $2\frac{1}{4}$ lbs), which will be adjusted depending on how you respond to the drug. You'll probably take the tablets once a day, though some people have the dose split between morning and evening and occasionally the drug is taken on alternate days. The drug can take up to three months to work.

It's not a painkiller so continue to take your other drugs that provide symptom relief.

Side-effects

These include succumbing to infections more often, because the drug suppresses the bone marrow, rashes, slight nausea, bruising more easily and liver problems. It can also make your red blood cells look large, but this isn't a problem.

To avoid or lessen some of these side-effects, try the following. Take it with or after food to prevent nausea. Try to avoid anyone who has an infection, and see your doctor if you keep getting sore throats or fevers. If you've not had chickenpox, try to avoid anyone with this or shingles. If you do come into contact with someone suffering from either of these, see your doctor in case special treatment is needed.

If you take the drug for a long time, it can slightly increase the risk of lymphomas (cancer of the lymph system, which is made up of the lymph glands, liver, spleen and bone marrow), though this is very rare. Symptoms would include unusual fevers and enlarged lymph glands. It's not a good idea to take the drug if you've had lymphomas in the past.

Poor kidney function can make the drug more powerful because it's not flushed out of the body, so you're unlikely to be put on this drug if your kidneys aren't working properly.

Azathioprine and other medicines

It can interact with some other drugs, so make sure your doctor knows what other drugs you take and check what over-the-counter products you can safely take. If you're taking the blood-thinning drug warfarin, it's unlikely you'll be given azathioprine. Drugs used for gout treatment can also interact with this drug. It doesn't affect the contraceptive pill.

Monitoring

Before going on the drug you'll have a full blood count done as well as liver function tests. Once you're on the drug you'll normally have monthly checks for eight weeks and then, if all is well, three-monthly checks.

Pregnancy

Don't become pregnant while taking azathioprine. You need to stop taking it three months before you start trying for a baby, using contraception during this time. If you do conceive while taking it, though, don't take your next dose and see your doctor as soon as possible.

Breastfeeding

Don't breastfeed while taking this drug.

Fertility

It is not known whether or not it affects men's sperm count, and it may slightly reduce fertility in women.

If you forget to take your tablets

Don't worry – just carry on as normal the next day. If you're on a divided dose and forget your morning tablet, you can take it any time up to midday, but, after this, just take your evening tablet as normal.

Flare-ups

Talk to your doctor about possible options. You may find that increasing your NSAID dose if there's scope is sufficient or you may need steroids. If you keep getting flare-ups you may need to change your drugs.

Vaccinations

Avoid live ones, opting for dead vaccines if possible.

Alcohol

Azathioprine can damage the liver, so check with your doctor how much you can safely drink.

Penicillamine

Penicillamine (the brand usually prescribed is Distamine) is rarely a drug of first choice. Doctors have different views about its usefulness. It can have similar side-effects to those of gold and may also cause muscle weakness problems. You probably won't be prescribed this drug unless you've had problems with other drugs, but it worked well for Sue.

'I started on penicillamine in 1995 after trying various other drugs, including methotrexate, which I didn't get on very well with. I was on penicillamine for a couple of years and it was wonderful. I could get up in the morning much more easily and go out shopping again. But it stopped working for me after the birth of my fourth child when I became very stiff and my joints became badly swollen.'

What to expect

It's taken in tablet form and a daily starting dose of 125 mg or 250 mg is normally given. For the first fortnight, you'll be asked to look out for rashes and mouth ulcers. If you develop an itchy, eczema-like rash during this time you may not be able to stay on the drug.

If all is well, the dose is increased – for example, from 125 mg to 250 mg, or 250 mg to 375 mg. The dose can be gradually increased to 1,000 mg (1 gram), but the evidence seems to be that there's no point increasing the dose if it doesn't work for you at 500 mg. Most people on the drug take a 500-mg dose, though some people find a 375-mg dose works for them.

It needs to be taken on an empty stomach at least an hour before food because some of the minerals in foods can affect absorption of the drug. The tablets can be taken all at once or may be split between morning and evening. It takes three months or so to work.

It's not a painkiller, so remember to keep taking your other drugs that provide symptom relief.

Side-effects

You may develop a muscle weakness disorder that mimics or looks like myasthenia gravis. This is a very rare side-effect, but it's serious, so, if it occurs, you'll need to come off the drug.

You may also temporarily lose your sense of taste for some

months, which can be rather frightening if you're not prepared for it. If your sense of taste hasn't returned after three months, your doctor may reduce the dose, but, if it still doesn't return then, you may need to stop taking the drug.

You need to ring your GP or rheumatology clinic within 48 hours if mouth ulcers start to develop because these could herald the start of a toxic drug reaction in your body, which means you need to come off the drug.

Other problems include bruising easily because of a low platelet count and susceptibility to infections because of a low white count. Let your doctor know as soon as possible if you're suffering more infections than before (sore throats, fevers and so on), kidney complications or a nasty blistering rash called pemphigus or other rashes. The drug can also temporarily cause another autoimmune disease called lupus (damaged and inflamed muscles, joints and various organs).

There aren't any known cancer risks attached to this drug at the moment.

The drug is derived from penicillin, so, if you're allergic to this, you should make sure your doctor knows. However, the drug can usually still be safely taken by people who are allergic to penicillin.

Penicillamine and other medicines

It's not usually prescribed with other DMARDs and some other types of medicines can also interact with the drug. Iron, zinc and antacids can reduce absorption of the drug, so check with your doctor or the pharmacist what you should do if you need to take a mineral supplement or an antacid. It doesn't affect the contraceptive pill.

Monitoring

A full blood count and urine checks are done, usually fortnightly for around six weeks, then at monthly intervals.

A blood test to check how well your kidneys are functioning isn't necessarily done routinely, though it may be a good idea to have one. A trace of protein in the urine indicates that the kidneys may not be working so well and further kidney tests may then be carried out. If there is a problem, the dose may be halved or you may need to stop taking the drug.

Pregnancy

It's best to come off the drug and then have a three-month gap before trying to conceive. If you do accidentally become pregnant while still taking the drug, you shouldn't worry, but don't take your next dose and get advice straight away about your position.

> Sue was on this drug when she found out she was 14 weeks pregnant (most potential damage to the baby would occur in the first three months of pregnancy). Most women don't have symptoms in pregnancy but Sue did and when her doctor tried to wean her off the drug, she had bad symptoms. She ended up staying on a half dose throughout her pregnancy and had a healthy baby.

Breastfeeding

The usual advice is not to breastfeed when you're taking this drug.

Fertility

The drug isn't thought to affect male or female fertility.

If you forget to take your tablets

Don't double up your next day's dose – just continue as normal.

Flare-ups

Options include increasing your NSAID dose, if there's scope, or to have steroid treatment. Alternatively, your doctor may increase the penicillamine dose – say, from 500 mg to 750 mg, though, as noted earlier, there's not much evidence that it's of benefit to go over 500 mg.

Vaccinations

Avoid live ones, having dead vaccines if possible.

Alcohol

There shouldn't be any particular problems with drinking alcohol, but check what you can safely drink with your doctor.

Cyclosporin (immunosuppressant)

This drug is used to prevent organ rejection in transplant operations, but it's now licensed for use as a treatment for rheumatoid arthritis.

It suppresses the immune system and works by blocking the action of the cytokines, which promote inflammation.

It doesn't necessarily work that well for rheumatoid arthritis and has some nasty side-effects, so doctors have different views about its usefulness. It's more powerful than azathioprine, but it's also a toxic drug. One of the brands commonly prescribed is Neoral. The drug may be used on its own or to boost the effectiveness of another disease-modifying drug.

What to expect

Tests include a full blood count and urine checks. If the results of the urine tests aren't normal, a blood test is done to check kidney function in more detail. Your blood pressure will also be checked and you'll be weighed.

If the test results are normal, you'll be prescribed the drug. The dose you're given is weight-related – 2.5 mg per kilo (about $2\frac{1}{4}$ lbs), with an average starting dose of 150 mg. It's usually split into a morning and evening dose to reduce nausea problems, though it can be taken all at once.

The drug isn't a painkiller so you need to keep taking your other drugs for symptom relief, but see below, under the heading Cyclosporin and other medicines, about NSAIDs.

You'll be asked to come back probably a fortnight later for a check-up. If there are any changes in kidney function and blood pressure, further tests may be needed. If there is a problem, the dose may be halved or you may need to come off the drug. If all is well, the dose will be increased.

The drug can take up to three months to start to work.

Side-effects

These include kidney problems, raised blood pressure, bruising easily, getting more infections than before, nausea, diarrhoea, gum problems and tiredness. If you've not had chickenpox before, try to avoid anyone with this or shingles. If you do come into contact with someone suffering from either of these illnesses, see your doctor in case special treatment is needed.

The drug quite often causes excessive facial and body hair to grow. There's no way of preventing this side-effect, so you need to keep removing the excess hair or stop taking the drug.

It does carry an increased risk of skin cancers and lymphomas, though these are more likely to occur when the drug is used for transplant patients and psoriasis. It's unclear what the cancer risk is if you're taking the drug as a treatment for rheumatoid arthritis, so check with your doctor how this slight risk of cancer relates to you.

The drug can also affect the liver, so it is unlikely to be suitable for you if you've got severe liver disease.

Cyclosporin and other medicines

It interacts with various drugs, including some antibiotics, antifungal and antiepileptic drugs, so find out what drugs can be safely taken with cyclosporin. NSAIDs can make kidney damage slightly more likely, so check with your doctor whether or not you can continue to take one of these drugs and at what dose.

It also interacts with the combined contraceptive pill and progestogen-only pill. Both still work, but the interaction between the two drugs can make cyclosporin levels rise, which could result in liver and kidney problems. So, if you really need to be on this drug, you may not be able to keep taking the pill. Discuss this with your doctor.

Note: There is an interaction between grapefruit juice and cyclosporin – the drug may not work so well if, for instance, you drink very large amounts of grapefruit juice each day. Eating a grapefruit every so often shouldn't be a problem, but, if you have large amounts of grapefruit juice each day, cut down or change to something else, such as apple juice. Double-check the position with your doctor.

Monitoring

Regular checks are usually done monthly after the first fortnight.

Pregnancy

You need to come off the drug at least three months before trying to become pregnant.

Breastfeeding

Don't breastfeed on this drug because very low levels of it easily pass into breast milk, though experience suggests problems are unlikely. There are two reports of mothers who breastfed while taking the drug and the babies appear to have suffered no harm.

Fertility

It doesn't appear to affect male or female fertility.

If you forget to take your tablets

Don't double up the next day's dose to compensate for the dose you missed, just take your next dose when it's due.

Flare-ups

Discuss the options for how to deal with these with your doctor.

Vaccinations

Avoid live vaccines and ask for dead ones, if possible.

Alcohol

Check with your doctor how much you can safely drink.

Cyclophosphamide (immunosuppressant)

This is a very powerful drug that is not commonly used for, and not that effective in, the treatment of rheumatoid arthritis.

It works by dampening down the immune system, reducing cell turnover and blocking the development of new cells.

Cyclophosphamide is an anti-cancer drug, but it's also occasionally prescribed in the treatment of rheumatoid arthritis. It's mainly used if there are no other alternatives for complications of rheumatoid arthritis, such as vasculitis, when they don't respond to steroid treatment.

It's also used to save eyesight if you get scleromalacia – a serious complication of scleritis, which is inflammation of the sclera (the white outer coat of the eye). The condition affects less than 1 per cent of people with rheumatoid arthritis.

It's normally used as a short-term treatment, for several months at most.

What to expect

You'll be very carefully monitored on this drug. It's available in tablet form, but is more commonly prescribed as an injection into the vein as an intravenous infusion, which is when the drug is slowly fed into the body. Your doctor will decide how often you need infusions.

Each infusion needs to be done in hospital and takes perhaps an hour. As it can damage the bladder, you need to drink lots of fluid – around 3 litres (5½ pints) – to protect your bladder. You also need to drink lots of fluid regularly if you're taking tablets. In order to further protect the bladder, a drug called Mesna is sometimes used when the cyclophosphamide is taken.

The drug can take around six weeks or so to work, depending on what problem it's being used to treat.

Side-effects

Nausea is a side-effect, though an anti-sickness pill can be taken to prevent this. Bruising easily, temporary hair loss, a rash, as well as, possibly, pins and needles in the hands and feet may also be experienced. It's more likely than the other DMARDs to suppress the bone marrow, so two weeks after the infusion a full blood test is done to check the white count.

If you've not had chickenpox before, avoid anyone with this or shingles. See the doctor if you do come into contact with someone who has one or other of these as you may need special treatment.

There's also a tiny risk of skin cancer with this drug, so check what the risk is for you when cyclophosphamide is used to treat your rheumatoid arthritis.

As discussed above, it can also damage the bladder, so it's very important to tell your doctor if you notice blood in your urine, in which case the drug dose may be altered.

It's not suitable for anyone who is pregnant or wanting to become pregnant, and isn't usually given to young girls unless there's no alternative (see under Fertility below).

Cyclophosphamide and other medicines

It's very important that everyone knows you're taking this drug because it can interact with various others. It doesn't interact with the contraceptive pill, though.

Monitoring

You'll be monitored very closely while you take this drug. Practice varies, but it's common to do a full blood count two weeks after the infusion or wait and do a blood count just before the next infusion. Infusions normally are given monthly.

Pregnancy

Check with your doctor, but you need to come off this drug usually around three to six months before you try for a baby and take precautions to avoid becoming pregnant during this time.

Breastfeeding

Don't breastfeed while taking this drug.

Fertility

The drug can lower the sperm count in men. In women, it can make periods stop and, if you have enough of it, the drug can bring on an early menopause. However, as it's only used as a short-term treatment at lower doses in the treatment of rheumatoid arthritis, there are fewer worries about its effects on fertility than when it is used to treat other health problems. Despite this, as it may damage the ovaries, some doctors co-prescribe the contraceptive pill with it to try and protect the ovaries.

Vaccinations

Avoid live vaccines and only have dead ones, if possible.

Alcohol

Check how much you can safely drink with your doctor.

Chlorambucil (immunosuppressant)

This is another anti-cancer drug. It reduces cell turnover and affects the immune system, but it's rarely used for rheumatoid arthritis treatment these days. However it is included here because it may be used if someone develops amyloidosis, which is when there is a protein deposit in various organs that causes the affected organ to become enlarged. This problem can occur in people who have a chronic disease such as rheumatoid arthritis, with just under 1 per cent of sufferers developing amyloidosis after they've had rheumatoid arthritis for some time. The good news is that, as rheumatoid arthritis treatments have improved because of the use of DMARDs, amyloidosis is less likely to occur as a complication of the disease today than was the case in the past.

Other treatments for amyloidosis are cyclophosphamide, though it's not that good a treatment for this, or steroids or azathioprine.

The drug can also help the joints.

Key points

You take a daily tablet. It can suppress the bone marrow and, with long-term use, there's a slightly increased risk of lymphomas and skin cancers. Regular checks, usually on a monthly basis, are done, including a full blood count and liver function tests.

Combination therapy

There are various reasons for taking several DMARDs together. Some hospitals in the past have done this, each drug being taken at a lower dose, as a way of trying to quickly control the disease. The rationale for this is that, as it's difficult to know in advance which drug will work for which patient and because the drugs are slow to work, it makes sense to use several drugs all at once.

Examples of combinations used at the start of treatment include low doses of methotrexate, azathioprine and hydroxychloroquine, or sulphasalazine, methotrexate and hydroxychloroquine.

Some studies have looked at this approach, but with conflicting results. For instance, in one trial with 209 patients, azathioprine plus methotrexate wasn't any better at slowing down the disease than azathioprine on its own or methotrexate on its own.

However, in another two-year-long study of 102 patients, triple therapy using methotrexate, plus sulphasalazine and hydroxychloroquine seemed to be better than sulphasalazine and hydroxychloroquine or methotrexate on its own, and triple therapy was no more toxic. Of patients given triple therapy, 77 per cent improved by at least 50 per cent, compared to 40 per cent of those taking sulphasalazine and hydroxychloroquine, and 33 per cent of those taking only methotrexate (*Drug and Therapeutics Bulletin*, 1998).

The usual way that you end up taking several of these drugs together is when a drug is added in to help a drug that is no longer working so well for you. For example, as discussed earlier, hydroxychloroquine is sometimes taken with methotrexate to prevent nodules developing.

Some clinics do still use combination therapy at the start of treatment. This isn't often done, but, if it's suggested and you're worried about what sort of side-effects you might have, don't be frightened to get more information. Ask why this is necessary, what side-effects you may experience if several drugs are taken together and discuss alternatives.

Bear in mind that your doctor may have good reason for wanting to start you on several drugs all at once. For instance, if you have liver disease the doctor knows that the most effective dose of a particular drug can't be used because you'd suffer side-effects if you took that much of it.

5

Steroids

Corticosteroids – or simply steroids as they're commonly called – are powerful anti-inflammatory drugs and, in a sense, are the equivalent of all the other drugs rolled into one. They were first used to treat rheumatic diseases around 50 years ago.

There were great expectations that these drugs could revolutionize the treatment of inflammatory diseases such as rheumatoid arthritis, but this enthusiasm turned to concern as it became clear over time that the drugs can have serious side-effects. Rheumatologists have different views about the place these drugs should have in the treatment of the disease. Some think that the drugs are valuable when used together with a slower-acting DMARD to quickly suppress the disease and prevent early damage. Other doctors think that the benefits of the drugs are not so great when the disadvantages of the drugs are taken into account.

Despite these concerns, many doctors think steroids are very useful drugs. The drugs act as painkillers, damp down inflammation and there's evidence that they can affect the disease process itself, and reduce the damage it does to the joints.

The drugs are similar to the natural corticosteroid hormones produced by the outer layer of the adrenal glands. These are two small glands situated on top of the kidneys and they secrete hormones directly into the bloodstream.

One of these is a very important hormone called cortisol, which suppresses inflammatory reactions in the body. Steroid drugs such as hydrocortisone or methylprednisolone mimic the action of this hormone.

Don't confuse the steroids we're talking about here with anabolic steroids – these are totally different drugs based on the male sex hormones and best known as body-building drugs.

Steroids work quickly and make you feel generally much better. They have the same effect as NSAIDs, but work in a different way and, unlike NSAIDs, steroids affect your immune system because they reduce the release and activity of white blood cells, which means you're more likely to fall prey to infections. Despite this, they play a central role in many people's treatment.

Jane was diagnosed as having rheumatoid arthritis when she was 40, and her whole body is affected by the disease. She's been on various drugs, but now takes a NSAID plus steroid tablets – four 1-mg tablets – that she takes all together at lunchtime. 'The steroids have helped the arthritis enormously. I probably wouldn't be able to get around without them. I also occasionally have a steroid injection when I'm in dire need, but I know the drugs can cause problems and the steroids may have had something to do with the heart attack I've had.'

Helen's symptoms started ten years ago when she was 46. Gold worked well for her, but she was taken off it because doctors mistakenly thought the disease was under control. It wasn't and when she was put back on gold it no longer worked for her. Since then, she's tried all sorts of other drugs without a lot of success. 'I'm in a lot of pain and I feel trapped sometimes because I can't turn over in bed. The only time I feel fit is when I have a steroid injection, for instance before I go on holiday or to tide me over Christmas, and the effects usually last around three months. I've also had a 14-day course of steroid tablets, which was brilliant – I couldn't believe the difference the tablets made. I need these drugs sometimes. I don't always like taking them, but there's only so much pain you can put up with.'

Mary, 54, has always been worried about the drug treatments for rheumatoid arthritis. She saw her father struggle with the disease and how cortisone affected him when he was given the drug in the 1950s. 'He became moon-faced, overweight and he was buried when he was 56. The secondary cause of death was the drug treatment.' For years she just took a NSAID, 'but I became quite poorly. I couldn't lift my hands to wash my hair and my shoulders were very painful and I had problems turning over in bed.' She reluctantly went on to gold and found that it worked for her for a time and that she suffered no side-effects. But, with various changes in her life, she started to go downhill again. She was put on methotrexate with folic acid, but had awful bowel problems with this and ended up in hospital. She is now taking a short-term course of steroid tablets and a painkiller occasionally. 'I do worry about steroids because of what happened to my father and I have to battle with my weight all the time. But the drugs do help and my wrists, elbows, shoulders, knees and ankles seem all right at the moment, though I've got some pain in my left knee.'

How steroids are used

In practice, the drugs are used in various ways and may be taken together with a painkiller and a NSAID and a DMARD on a temporary, or sometimes longer-term, basis.

They're mainly used in the following situations:

- when you've been newly diagnosed to give rapid relief when you're waiting for the DMARD to start to work;
- to make you feel better generally;
- to damp down joint stiffness due to joint inflammation;
- to quickly settle a flare-up.

If you're going on holiday and have had problems with flare-ups previously while away, an intramuscular steroid injection given just before you go can be a good way to prevent this. Alternatively, it can be useful sometimes to take a low-dose course of steroid tablets with you on holiday in case you have problems.

Steroids may also be used to give symptom relief if you've got active disease and you can't take a DMARD because you're trying for a baby.

Steroids may also be used to treat various complications of the disease, such as vasculitis, eye disease and, less commonly, for a type of anaemia that occurs when certain antibodies attack the red blood cells, as well as inflammation of the lining of the heart.

What to expect

The drugs can give rapid relief, within two to three days, sometimes sooner. Steroids are prescribed in the following ways.

Tablets

The most common way for the drug to be taken is in tablet form, and the steroid most commonly prescribed is prednisolone. Low-dose steroid tablets – that is, between 5 and 10 mg a day – are often used long term together with a DMARD or sometimes on their own.

The dose is normally taken once a day, with or after food to minimize stomach problems. Taken this way, the steroid can be very effective for many people. Indeed, most people respond to the low dose, which can be a welcome relief after years of pain.

People who have rheumatoid arthritis are normally very sensitive to steroids and respond to low-dose treatment – that is, 5 or 7.5 mg or, at most, 10 mg daily – which means side-effects are less likely than with the higher doses. If a 10-mg dose doesn't help, it's unlikely that you will respond to a higher dose than this.

Note: Don't be alarmed if you need to take a higher-dose tablet for non-joint problems, such as vasculitis (see below) or inflammation of the lining of the heart (also a 30–40-mg dose), because it's usually just for a short time.

Tablets are also used to treat vasculitis. You'll be put on a high dose – perhaps 30–40 mg. When the vasculitis is under control, you'll come off the steroid, though, sometimes, you may need to stay on a low-dose steroid tablet to prevent recurrence of the vasculitis.

A dose of around 50–60 mg is used to treat the serious eye disease scleromalacia, also discussed below.

Intravenous injection

This is given at a hospital outpatient clinic and occasionally on an in-patient basis. Methylprednisolone is the drug normally used, and it is injected into the vein. However, intravenous injections aren't used that much because they're more impractical than the other options and they do carry risks. This said, it is possible you might have an intravenous injection if you have vasculitis though even in this case tablets are normally given, as discussed above.

An intravenous injection may also be given perhaps with cyclophosphamide if you develop a serious eye complication, such as scleromalacia (mentioned in the last chapter under the heading Cyclophosphamide). You will recall that in this the sclera – the white outer part of the eye – becomes constantly inflamed, red and very sore and so thin that it may perforate in the worst cases. Here, too, it's more usual to give very high dose tablets (50–60-mg steroid doses), as discussed above. Nevertheless, an infusion can be given and sometimes an infusion plus tablets are used.

Intramuscular injection

Usually a 120-mg steroid dose is given, which seems high, but a slow-release preparation is used (see under the heading Summary of steroid preparations later in this chapter) so you actually get about 5 mg a day.

The dose is injected into the buttock and shouldn't hurt. This option is used to settle a flare-up quickly and help stiff joints.

Intra-articular injections (joint injections)

Inflamed joints are often treated in this way, particularly if you're having problems with one or two joints. However, it's impractical to inject all joints. The dose is normally 40 mg.

It can be given with a local anaesthetic so ask about this if you've had pain with a previous injection.

The joints often injected are the knees, ankles, elbows, shoulders, finger joints, knuckles and wrists. The hips are not because giving lots of injections there can lead to crumbling of the hip bones.

> Pat, 47, who has had the disease for ten years, has had some joint injections in the last few years. One of her knees becomes very swollen, and the injection is given after the fluid has been drained off. Both ankles also get quite swollen, so these are also injected. 'The injections work almost straight away and have been very helpful. They used to last for about three months, but unfortunately the last one had an effect for only about six weeks.'

Side-effects aren't usual. You may feel a bit achy for the rest of the day after the injection and, if you can, it's a good idea to rest for 24 hours or so.

Injections are invasive procedures and, although it happens very rarely, it's possible that an injection could introduce an infection into the joint. If your joint becomes hot and painful, then see your doctor straight away.

If you take the blood-thinning drug warfarin, your rheumatologist may want you to have thicker blood at the time of the injection because you'll bleed more easily if the needle scrapes the inside of the joint. Your warfarin dose may therefore need to be temporarily reduced.

There isn't an upper limit to the number of injections you can have into a joint, but it's not a good idea to have them on a regular basis – for instance, every two months – because of the risk of joint damage. Also, frequent problems with a joint are a sign that the disease isn't being adequately controlled and so your doctor will want to look at the overall management of your problems. This can be tricky, though. For instance, you may be doing well generally on sulphasalazine, but have one joint that keeps playing up. The question is whether the sulphasalazine dose should be increased, though this might lead to more side-effects, or to give you joint injections more frequently with the risks this involves.

Soft tissue injections

These are injections into painful, inflamed tissue near a joint. For instance, the area around the wrist can be injected in cases of carpal tunnel syndrome, which is when the nerve in the wrist is being squeezed by the inflamed joint lining of the wrist bones. Tendon sheaths can also be injected. You may notice a flattening of the skin or it being whiter around the injection area.

Summary of steroid preparations

To recap, prednisolone is the drug most often prescribed if you're taking tablets.

Methylprednisolone is most often prescribed if you're having intramuscular, intravenous or intra-articular injections, as this drug is a slow-release one because of the metal in it. It's also stronger than hydrocortisone – one of the other preparations used for joint injections (triamcinolone is another one).

Don't be afraid to ask about the various steroid treatments so that you get the best one for you.

Side-effects

What's best for you in your particular case involves weighing up the benefits of these drugs against their disadvantages, but side-effects are more likely the longer you're on steroids and the higher the dose you're taking. It's often assumed that injections are safer than tablets, but this isn't necessarily so.

Intramuscular injections

Not a lot is known about the side-effects of this type of injection. If you have one of these occasionally or once a year, there shouldn't be anything to worry about. If you're having them regularly, however – say, three-monthly intramuscular injections – you may be more vulnerable to side-effects.

Joint and soft tissue injections

These have local side-effects in the injection area. Also, tiny amounts of the drug get into the circulation, but this isn't a problem for most people. However, if you've got diabetes, you need to be aware of this (see also the point below on diabetes under the heading Short-term side-effects). It's also possible that, if you have frequent joint injections, the steroid may destroy cartilage and lead to earlier development of osteoarthritis and also, possibly, localized thinning of the bones.

Short-term side-effects

These include the following.

- Some people develop a peculiar metallic taste, though this is unlikely on low-dose tablets and more likely a result of intravenous treatment or higher doses. It's a temporary side-effect that is related particularly to higher doses, but, as you shouldn't be on one for long, this shouldn't be too much of a problem.
- Steroid tablets can disrupt your body clock so that you start to wake up in the middle of the night.
- The tablets can make your stomach a bit sore.
- You'll feel much better generally and less tired and lethargic.
- You'll probably feel hungry all the time because the steroids increase your appetite.
- It's also possible you'll put on weight due to retaining more fluid in your body.
- Problems such as asthma and bronchitis may improve.
- Heart failure may worsen due to fluid retention.
- If you have diabetes, you may find it gets worse because steroids slightly raise blood sugar, so your treatment may need adjustment. Even an occasional injection can affect your blood sugar, so don't panic, and be more vigilant about doing your diabetic checks and, if in doubt about anything, see your doctor.
- Steroid-induced diabetes.
- Blood pressure could rise because of fluid retention.

Long-term side-effects from long-term treatment

Long-term effects include those described below.

- Steroids can cause osteoporosis (the bone-thinning disease). Bone density scans can be done to check the state of your bones. Probably the best scan at the moment is the dual energy X-ray absorptiometry scan – DEXA for short. Drug treatments for osteoporosis include HRT as well as non-hormonal bisphosphonate drugs, such as cyclical etidronate (Didronel) or alendronate (Fosamax). Rheumatologists may have different views about how to prevent problems if you're taking steroids. For example, some may ask you to take calcium supplements routinely or you may be given one of the bisphosphonates.
- Increased risk of infections.
- Increased risk of cataracts.
- Increased sensitivity to the sun, so you may develop skin rashes.
- Slight wasting of the muscles.
- Thinner skin.
- Mood changes are possible.
- Bruising easily because the drugs make the tissues fragile and leaky.
- Thinning hair.
- Children's growth can be stunted by long-term steroid treatment because the bones don't grow as well and the muscles can become a bit wasted. Ask if any of the steroid preparations are less likely to cause these problems. Deflazacort, for example, is very costly and perhaps not quite as good as prednisolone, but it's less likely to cause growth problems, so may be a better choice for children and teenagers. Discuss what options there are with the rheumatologist.

Who can take steroids?

Lots of people take steroids. They can be safely taken if you have some types of cancer or chronic bronchitis, but, because of their side-effects, they're not advisable for everyone.

- If you've got significant osteoporosis, the doctor will have to weigh up whether or not you should take steroids as the drugs cause thinning of the bones. As discussed above, your doctor will probably organize a DEXA bone density scan and give you a treatment for the condition.

- If you're already taking some steroid-based hormone treatment for other conditions, such as Addison's disease, your doctor will have to assess whether or not you can take a steroid for your rheumatoid arthritis or if this would be too problematical.
- You can take steroids if you've had an ulcer in the past because of the low doses normally used for the treatment of rheumatoid arthritis. Steroids are also not so toxic to the stomach as the NSAIDs. However, make sure your doctor knows about this. If you're on a higher dose temporarily, an antacid may be prescribed if you're suffering from a sore stomach. Some doctors may do this from the outset to avoid problems occurring.

Cautions

When you receive steroid treatment on a long-term basis, the drugs suppress the adrenal glands so that they don't produce steroid hormones. In times of acute stress (for instance, if you need an operation, have an accident or have a particularly nasty infection – maybe one that requires antibiotics), your body won't necessarily be able to produce enough extra cortisol – a very important corticosteroid hormone. In these situations, you'll need extra steroid treatment, so it's important to let everyone know that you're on steroids and carry a steroid warning card with you (see under Monitoring later in this chapter).

Don't suddenly stop taking steroids if you've been on them for more than several weeks because your adrenal glands won't be making enough cortisol and you'll suddenly be left short, which could be dangerous. If you need to come off a steroid drug, your doctor will gradually reduce the dose to allow your body time to start producing its own hormones again.

How to minimize the side-effects of steroids

Keep active to reduce thinning of the bones and wasting of the muscles. Try swimming to keep your muscles in good condition and do weight-bearing exercise, such as walking, on a regular basis to protect your bones. Ask your doctor how you can best help yourself. The self-help groups listed at the end of the book, such as the National Osteoporosis Society, provide lots of excellent information on this.

Steroids can disrupt your body clock, so it's best to take the drug in the morning as this will mean that there's less likelihood of waking up in the night.

You may find you get a sore stomach, so take your tablets with or after food.

The drugs will make you feel hungry, but try not to overeat.

Wear a sunblock in sunlight.

To reduce cataract formation, wear sunglasses that filter out the harmful rays, particularly UVB. Some research suggests that a diet high in antioxidants, such as vitamins E and C, can prevent the eye damage done by unstable chemicals produced in the body called free radicals, though some doctors are sceptical about this. It's a good idea, none the less, to have a wholesome diet rich in fresh fruit and vegetables that will give you plenty of vitamin C and ensure a good supply of vitamin E by eating nuts, wheatgerm and dark green vegetables.

Be vigilant about avoiding people with infections because you're more vulnerable to catching them. For example, you'll be more susceptible to developing a chest infection after having a cold. See your doctor if you're worried you're developing something.

Chickenpox is a common infection that people think of as trivial, but it can be dangerous for anyone on long-term steroid treatment. So, try to steer clear of children or adults who have it and see your doctor if you think you've come into contact with an infected person or that you're developing the infection. If you haven't had chickenpox before, your doctor might give you an inoculation that is made of antibodies from people who've had chickenpox, which will help you fight the infection if you catch it. Also try to avoid anyone who has shingles – a blistering painful rash over one part of the body, often the abdomen or chest and on one side of the trunk – because you can get chickenpox from someone with shingles as the chickenpox virus, herpes zoster, is responsible for both infections.

Be aware that steroids can mask the signs of inflammation that warn you that you have an infection, which may result in you not realizing that you have an infection until it's well advanced. If you get a fever, vomiting or diarrhoea, see your doctor and indeed if in any doubt about anything.

Steroids can temporarily induce diabetes that goes once you come off the steroids. If you've just started on steroids and notice you're more thirsty than previously and pass more urine, you could have raised blood sugar and it's important to see your doctor.

Steroids and other medicines

Steroids may interact with some other drugs and over-the-counter medicines, so double-check what you can safely take with your doctor and the pharmacist.

Steroids can be taken with NSAIDs and many other drugs, and won't affect the efficacy of the contraceptive pill. If you are on the pill, though, let your doctor know as it may make the steroids a bit more powerful.

Steroids can usually be taken with the blood-thinning drug warfarin. Make sure, though, that your rheumatologist knows you're taking it and also that the anticoagulation clinic knows you're on steroids as they may want to do additional blood checks.

Pregnancy

Steroids are safer to take than many of the other drugs discussed so far, though the general rule is that all drugs are best avoided during pregnancy. However, the usual advice is that you can become pregnant while taking steroids at the doses usually prescribed for this disease, but it's a good idea to discuss the exact position with your doctor when you're thinking about having a baby.

Breastfeeding

Steroids are excreted in small amounts in breast milk, but it's thought to be safe to breastfeed if you're on anything up to a 40–50-mg daily dose. Anything above this might affect the baby's health by suppressing the adrenal glands. Although the evidence is that higher doses aren't a significant risk, it's probably a good idea to avoid breastfeeding for three to four hours after taking your steroid dose. You can prepare for this by expressing breast milk and freezing it in the special bags available for this purpose.

If you've had a slow-release intramuscular 120-mg injection, this should be safe because it works out about 5 mg per day. Double-check what you should do with your doctor.

Fertility

Steroids shouldn't affect male or female fertility.

Monitoring

Checks aren't usually done if you're having an occasional intramuscular or intravenous injection. However, if you're on long-term treatment, various precautions are taken. When you start on steroids, you'll be given a steroid card with your details on it – name, address, the date you started on steroids, the dose and method of administration. Make sure you take this to all your clinic appointments and carry it with you at all other times. Some people wear steroid bracelets – ask your clinic if you want to know more about this.

Otherwise, there aren't any standard pre-steroid checks as there are for some of the other drugs, though, if you're at risk of osteoporosis or already have it, a DEXA scan will be carried out to measure bone density, as discussed earlier under Long-term side-effects. Regular blood tests aren't usually done either while you're on steroids, but you'll be having these anyway if you're taking a DMARD. This said, some doctors may do some checks from time to time, though practice varies on this. If you're on warfarin, more blood checks may be needed to make sure your blood doesn't get too thin.

If you're diabetic, you'll be asked to keep a close eye on yourself in the first couple of weeks after you've started taking steroids. If problems occur, you need to contact your diabetic clinic.

If you have had some heart failure you may notice that you become a bit more breathless, which may mean that your heart or blood pressure medicine needs to be increased.

If you forget to take your dose

As mentioned earlier it's important not to suddenly stop taking steroids because this can leave you short of important hormones. Check with your doctor what you should do in advance so that you're prepared and know what to do if this happens. The general advice is likely to be that, if you've been on steroids for three months or more on a 5-mg or greater dose, you should not worry too much if you miss one day, though you'll feel more tired. If you've missed two days, it's safe to double up the next day's dose. If you're on a morning dose and forget this, simply take it in the evening.

If you're vomiting a lot and think that you vomited up your morning tablet, try to take it later in the day. If you're unsure whether you brought up the tablet or not, it's still usually best to take another tablet and, in effect, have a double dose rather than none at all.

Vaccinations

Avoid live vaccines, opting for dead ones, if possible.

Alcohol

It's safe to have alcohol, but drink in moderation because, when you're on steroids, your stomach lining could be a bit sensitive.

6
New Treatment Developments and Drug Trials

At the time of writing, there are no drugs that can cure rheumatoid arthritis, but the new DMARD leflunomide (Arava) discussed in Chapter 4 holds much promise. Then there are the two new biological agents discussed below. The new drugs mean that there are more treatment options, and the more research that goes into drugs the greater the chance of finding a cure. Other therapies and approaches are also under development that may prove to be useful for some people with rheumatoid arthritis. Altogether, the future looks much brighter than ever before.

Biological agents

The two new drugs infliximab (Remicade) and etanercept (Enbrel) mentioned briefly in Chapter 4 are DMARDs that work in a different way and are also administered differently. However, they are likely to be very expensive at around £7,000 per person per year. This means that they're unlikely to be routinely available, perhaps only being used in large, specialist research centres, so may not be drugs of first choice. They may be used if you have moderate to severe problems and don't respond to the other DMARDs or can't take them because of their side-effects.

These drugs are genetically engineered biological agents that tackle the disease process in a new way. Both drugs disable inflammatory cytokines. Enbrel blocks the action of tumour necrosis factor. Remicade also blocks the action of tumour necrosis factor, but not in quite the same way. Trials of another biological agent are also in progress.

These drugs have been greeted with excitement by some clinicians, but it's a question of waiting to see how they work in practice. It's not quite clear how effective a drug can be if it just works to combat one part of the inflammatory process in what is a complicated disease.

Enbrel

This drug is licensed for treatment in the USA. In early 2000 it completed the licensing process in the UK and is now available.

There's not that much information available about this drug at the moment because it hasn't been in general use for long. It's possible to give some limited details about it, but you need to check what the latest information is with your rheumatologist.

In one trial with 69 patients who took the drug for 90 days, 74 per cent of patients showed profound, clinically important improvements. So far, the drug is described as being well tolerated – that is, people seem to have few problems when they take it.

What to expect

Enbrel can be taken by all age groups and the dose is likely to be a twice-weekly 25-mg subcutaneous dose self-injected just under the skin, probably into the buttock, though you may find self-injection difficult if you've got swollen, stiff fingers.

Check what time of day you should give yourself the injection. You may be advised to do this in the morning so you've got time to see your doctor for advice about what to do if you have a reaction.

In one trial with 782 patients, including 69 children, they were followed up for 33 months. Of these patients, 43 per cent of people taking the drug developed some sort of skin reaction around the injection area, but only four patients actually withdrew from treatment because of this. Don't panic if this happens to you, but, if the reaction is very bad, you may need to come off the drug. Explore if there are any ways round the problem with your doctor first.

Enbrel can take up to three months to start to work. It's licensed as a drug that can be used in its own right or as a helper – that is, together with another DMARD, such as methotrexate.

Side-effects

An itchy nettle-type rash (in the area of the injection or, perhaps, all over the body) is a possibility, though uncommon – a rash occurred in just one case in a study of 57 people taking the drug. If this happens, you need to get advice about whether or not you can continue with the injections.

The drug acts on the immune system in a slightly different way from the other drugs described earlier and there are concerns about whether or not it has any cancer risks – for example, whether or not lymphomas may develop. However, it's too early to have any answers to these concerns at the moment.

As the drug affects your immune system, you also need to double-check if you should be careful about avoiding people with infections such as chickenpox.

Enbrel and other medicines

Check with your doctor what medicines you can safely take with Enbrel. Also double-check what over-the-counter medicines you can safely have.

Pregnancy

Check the position on this, but the advice is probably the same as it is for other drugs – that is, you shouldn't become pregnant while taking it and need to stop taking it for a time before trying for a baby.

Breastfeeding

Check whether or not it's safe to breastfeed while on this drug.

Fertility

Ask your doctor if the drug affects male and female fertility in any way.

Flare-ups

The advice is likely to be the same as that for other DMARDs, but double-check with your doctor. If there's leeway, it may be possible to increase your NSAID dose or, if you're taking methotrexate, your doctor may increase the methotrexate dose if your body is coping with the drug.

Vaccinations

Again it's probably advisable to avoid live vaccines and have dead ones if possible, but double-check with your doctor.

Alcohol

It's probably safe to drink alcohol, but, again double-check with your doctor.

Remicade

There's not a great deal of information at the moment about this drug, as it is very new – it received a licence for the treatment of rheumatoid arthritis in the first half of 2000.

The information so far about it is that it's given by injection into the vein over a couple of hours every couple of months by a health professional. It'll probably be used together with methotrexate. Talk to your doctor for more information about this drug.

New NSAIDs

NSAIDs are very helpful, as discussed in Chapter 3, but they can have a number of side-effects because they act not only against the nasty type of COX-2 enzymes responsible for producing inflammatory prostaglandins, but also against the COX-1 enzymes responsible for making beneficial prostaglandins that protect the stomach. The result is that, as we saw, digestive problems and ulcers are a significant side-effect of these drugs.

For some time, drug companies have been developing drugs that just target the COX-2 enzymes and there are already drugs such as meloxicam (Mobic), discussed in Chapter 3, and etodolac (Lodine), that act more against COX-2 than COX-1.

Now there are two more drugs called COX-2-specific inhibitors that are meant to be kinder to the stomach and just work against COX-2. These are celecoxib (Celebrex) and rofecoxib (Vioxx). Celebrex is now available, having been licensed for rheumatoid arthritis and osteoarthritis in the UK in early 2000. Vioxx has already received a licence in the UK, but only for osteoarthritis.

As these drugs are supposed to damp down the nasty COX-2 enzymes but not interfere with COX-1 enzymes, they should have a good anti-inflammatory effect without causing stomach, asthma and kidney problems.

It's unclear yet how well these new drugs will work in the long term, though studies suggest they work as well as drugs such as diclofenac but cause fewer stomach problems. In practice, doctors will wait to see how these drugs work when they're widely used in the community.

Talk to your doctor about the possibility of trying this type of drug if you suffer from stomach upsets with the traditional NSAIDs. Note, however, that if you have a history of stomach or duodenal ulcers you'll probably be advised against taking these COX-2-specific inhibitors. It's also worth asking your doctor if it might be a good idea for you to try this type of drug if you have kidney problems that worsened when you took the older type of NSAID or if you have asthma or found that you suffered from dizziness on the older drugs.

Dose

Celebrex (celecoxib)

For rheumatoid arthritis, the dose is 100–200 mg twice a day, with a maximum daily dose of 400 mg. For osteoarthritis, the options include taking 100 mg morning and night, making 200 mg a day, or taking 200 mg morning and night, making 400 mg a day, or taking a single 200-mg daily dose.

Vioxx (rofecoxib)

For osteoarthritis one or two tablets are taken daily. They are each 12.5–25 mg. The tablets are best taken with food and aren't available in a slow-release form.

Drug interactions

Double-check what drugs can be safely taken with the COX-2-specific inhibitors. If you're taking the blood-thinning drug warfarin, you may not be able to take these newer NSAIDs. They shouldn't interact with the contraceptive pill, though.

Pregnancy

These drugs can be taken up to the first day of your missed period. Then, do not take them for the duration of your pregnancy.

Breastfeeding

It's best not to breastfeed while on these drugs, but check with your doctor.

Other approaches

Prosorba column

This therapy filters the blood. It involves removing blood, taking any rheumatoid factor antibodies out of it, then putting the purified blood back into the body. What's called a Prosorba column (absorbent material that removes the antibodies that are thought to cause the problem) is used with a technique called plasmapheresis

– sometimes known as plasma exchange – which is a way of removing or reducing the concentration of unwanted substances in the blood.

According to the Arthritis National Research Foundation in the USA – where the treatment has been recommended for moderate to severe rheumatoid arthritis – it's similar to the process used for kidney dialysis. Blood is removed from your arm and put through a machine that separates the blood cells from the plasma (the clear fluid part of blood). The plasma is then put through the Prosorba column and then put back with the blood cells and finally returned to you. The session takes place at a hospital and lasts around two hours. Standard treatment usually consists of weekly sessions for 12 weeks.

It's not clear how effective it is to purify the blood of these antibodies because they only account for one part of the inflammatory process. However, according to the Arthritis National Research Foundation, clinical trials in the USA found that nearly a half of those people who had failed to respond to drugs such as methotrexate showed significant clinical improvement after going through this therapy, and the benefit lasted up to 75 weeks for some people.

Another overview of studies so far commented that there is limited information at the moment, but that blood filtration using the Prosorba column may decrease symptoms in about one in three people who aren't helped by the other drugs or suffer side-effects from them. In one study, improvements generally happened only after the 12 treatments had finished.

The treatment can cause its own side-effects, such as a temporary increase in swelling of the joints, as well as pain and fatigue after treatment. Other side-effects include fever, chills, low blood pressure and nausea.

The treatment isn't advisable for anyone with vasculitis and certain blood conditions. Also, if you are taking an ACE inhibitor, which is used to treat high blood pressure, you need to stop taking it for at least 72 hours before starting the treatment.

A lot of questions still need to be answered about this therapy. For instance, how often would you need retreatment, how well does the method work in the longer term and can other DMARDs be given if you're treated with this method? It's a costly treatment because it involves visits to hospital each time.

Ask your rheumatologist for the latest information on this if you want to find out more.

Collagen

Cartilage is made up in part of collagen and so research is under way that is looking into whether or not collagen tablets made from animal sources can help arthritis sufferers.

Collagen is a tough, fibrous protein that is an important part of bones, tendons and connective tissue as it holds together the various structures in the body. The idea behind collagen therapy is to make the immune system more tolerant of cartilage so that the body doesn't attack it.

These tablets may have a place in the treatment of osteoarthritis or the secondary osteoarthritis that can develop later on with rheumatoid arthritis. However, as cartilage destruction isn't the root of the problem in rheumatoid arthritis (collagen is not part of the joint lining), it's unclear how helpful these tablets are for this disease. The rationale behind using collagen tablets for rheumatoid arthritis may be that it's important to protect the cartilage because, if it's attacked, it could start off the inflammatory process in the joint lining, though there's no strong evidence for this. So, it's not clear how collagen would affect the autoimmune aspect of rheumatoid arthritis, but it's possible that if you take collagen you might suffer less secondary osteoarthritis later on.

Collagen products are sold in some health shops. It's important to keep taking your normal drugs if you decide to try a supplement and it shouldn't interact with them. If you're interested in taking collagen, it's a good idea to discuss this with your rheumatologist to see what the advice is about the usefulness of this approach for you.

Bone marrow stem cell transplants

The idea here is to destroy and wipe out those cells in the immune system that have been programmed to destroy joints in the hope that new cells produced in the bone marrow will not attack the joints. However, it's a very risky experimental procedure and in 8 per cent of cases the patient does not survive it. Again, talk to your doctor if you want more information on this, but bear in mind that it's highly experimental.

Monoclonal antibodies

There's experimental research into chemically made antibodies that will disable the antibodies that destroy the joints. Treatment is given by intravenous injection in hospital.

As this treatment fundamentally alters the immune system, the risk of developing certain tumours and lymphomas may increase and there's a greater risk of infections.

Drug trials

All new drugs have to go through a costly, lengthy research process that can last many years before they can be licensed for use. This procedure is designed to find out whether or not the drugs are safe to take and if they're beneficial.

Drugs go through various stages. First, they have to be tested on animals before they can be tested on people. If the drug gets through the animal trials, it's then tested on people in three phases.

In Phase I trials, which usually last up to two years, a small number of healthy volunteers are given the drug so that doctors can find out how safe different doses of it are, plus its risks and side-effects, and how it interacts with other drugs.

In Phase II trials, which can last around a couple of years, the drug is used on 100 or more patients to see if it works as it's meant to.

Phase III trials are much bigger – over a thousand patients take part and the trials may last around four years. The drug is tested in more detail to see how well it works for this larger group of people. The new drug will be compared with existing drugs or a placebo (a dummy pill). However, nowadays it's not justified to give no treatment, so it's more likely that participants will be on either an established existing drug treatment or the drug under investigation and observed, usually for six months to a year.

A double-blind trial is organized, which is when neither doctors nor patients know which drug is being taken. Only the drug company has this information until the trial has been completed. The code is then cracked and this information is given to participants and medical staff.

It's at the Phase III stage, when the drug has already gone through various safety tests, that you might be asked whether or not you want to take part in a trial.

Drug companies are normally looking for people who've only had the disease for a couple of years and who've only tried about two of the other DMARDs. So you're more likely to be asked if you've been recently diagnosed with the disease than if you're a long-term sufferer.

Points to consider

Drugs do eventually need to be tested on human beings. If you volunteer to take part, the drug you help test may benefit you or others, but there is an element of risk because the side-effects aren't fully known at this stage even though the drug will by now have been through rigorous safety testing procedures. On the other hand, you are closely monitored, which some people see as a benefit, and if you have a flare-up, you'll be seen very quickly.

If you're doing well on your present medicines, you need to discuss if it makes sense to change things. For instance, if you're doing well on a DMARD and come off it to take part in the trial, will it work for you if you go back on it at a later date? (This last question is discussed in Chapter 4 under the heading The choice of drugs.)

Questions to ask

If you're interested, check what other drugs you can take while you're on the trial. You'll normally be allowed to take your NSAIDs though not alter the dose, plus a painkiller when you need it. You may have to come off any steroid you're taking three months before you start on the trial. The conditions, usually, are that you can continue to take the steroid if you stay on the same dose, but not if you take it on an irregular basis.

You would be wise to check how often tests are done and which ones will be carried out.

Ask which drug the trial drug is being compared to as you need to let the doctor know if you've previously been on that drug and had problems with it.

Ask what's known about the side-effects of the study drug so far.

If you're asked to take part in a drug trial, you're under no obligation to do so. If you're interested, you should be given time to think it over, not pressurized or hurried into making a decision, and you should be given information to read about the trial.

You'll be asked to sign a consent form if you do want to take part and you can pull out of the trial whenever you want. Some people fear that they'll be blacklisted if they do this, but there shouldn't be a problem. If there is, though, don't suffer in silence and ask to see a different consultant. Normally, the best way to do this is to talk to the rheumatology nurse or your GP.

STOP PRESS

Encouraging research results from a small-scale study of treatment carried out at University College London have been greeted with much excitement.

Treatment suppressed part of the immune system and aimed to destroy white cells – known as B cells because they can sometimes make rogue antibodies that attack the body – in the hope that new B cells manufactured by the body would produce normal antibodies.

Treatment consisted of a mix of drugs: rituximab (already used to treat lymphomas) to destroy the B cells, plus two other drugs, prednisolone and cyclophosphamide (already used in the treatment of rheumatoid arthritis, and talked about earlier in the book). Most of the 20 patients who took part in the study were reported to have benefited from the treatment, and an international trial is now under way.

Meanwhile it is important to be cautious about these early results and to adopt a wait and see policy. No firm conclusions can be drawn from a small-scale study involving just 20 people, and much more research is needed to establish the real value of this approach in terms of its effectiveness and side-effects, and whether it is risky to suppress the immune system in this way. The interest has been in rituximab, but it is also important to know what part prednisolone and cyclophosphamide played in improving symptoms.

7

Supplements and Other Approaches

You may want to try various supplements, make dietary changes or try complementary therapies in order to ease the discomfort of your rheumatoid arthritis symptoms. Some people say that approaches other than drug therapy have helped them, while others say they haven't noticed any benefit.

Sue says, 'I've tried garlic and fish oil, but they haven't helped me. All I know is that I can't drink red wine since my daughter was born last year as it really does aggravate my symptoms.'

Pat worries about the side-effects of conventional drugs. She has used supplements for some time, thinks they're helpful and that her need for drug treatment has reduced as a result of taking the supplements.

She was diagnosed with the disease ten years ago when she was in her late thirties and has two children aged fifteen and ten. She says, 'In terms of conventional medicines, I've had steroid injections for my ankles and one of my knees, which has been very swollen and keeps playing up. I also use painkillers and occasionally try ibuprofen if I'm very stiff, though I don't use it all the time because I find it gives me a very dry mouth and my bones feel brittle.

'For seven years I've taken evening primrose oil – 1,000 mg a day, which my GP prescribes for me. I think this has helped and that without it I'd have more deformed joints. In addition, I take a zinc and mineral supplement, which I get from the chemist. I also take a spoonful of cod liver oil a day, and a year ago I started to take one ginger and curcumin capsule a day, which I get from a health shop. I think it's helped because I don't take so many painkillers now. I've also been taking vitamin B_3 for about 18 months and I think this has helped my fingers, which used to be very stiff but are more supple now. If I can, I also drink nettle tea once a day as this is supposed to have an anti-inflammatory action.

'I think the drugs and other things I take can go together, and

I couldn't just rely on the supplements. I'm also aware that herbs and supplements aren't totally safe, so I try to spread out the doses and keep them to a minimum. I know my doctor wants me to go on methotrexate, but I don't want to do this at the moment unless it's absolutely necessary.'

Mary has tried various drugs and had problems with side-effects. 'I do worry about taking a cocktail of drugs. At the moment I'm taking a short-term course of steroid tablets and I have the occasional painkiller. I tried homeopathy for a year and I think it helped initially, but it doesn't seem to now. At the moment I feel all right, apart from one of my knees, and I'm pleased because a bone scan showed that my bones are in good condition and I'm not developing osteoporosis. But I'm a bit worried about what's going to happen. I've persisted trying to do it naturally with the homeopathy because I want to keep my body as healthy as possible, but I think I may need more drug treatment now. I'm worried about taking more steroids and the thought of taking another powerful drug worries me because of the bad time I had before with one of them.'

Can other approaches help?

Many people turn hopefully to other approaches because the conventional drugs don't or no longer work for them and/or they've suffered nasty side-effects.

Claims are made that some supplements can help in coping with arthritis and there are many anecdotal stories that other approaches can help, as in Pat's case. However, there's often a lack of hard scientific evidence at the moment to back this all up. There's also the added confusion that osteoarthritis and rheumatoid arthritis are often discussed as though they're one and the same thing, and that what works for one condition will work for the other. As discussed, these are two different conditions and if a supplement helps in osteoarthritis it doesn't follow that it'll necessarily help in rheumatoid arthritis. This doesn't mean you shouldn't try other approaches, but it's worth bearing in mind certain points discussed below.

Don't assume you can't talk to your doctors about wanting to try other things. Many doctors are more open-minded about these things than in the past and many are comfortable about the idea of patients taking supplements, other remedies or trying complementary therapies alongside conventional medicines. In fact, there is a strong move to integrate orthodox and complementary medicines so that people can get the best of both worlds. So, don't be scared to ask for your doctors' views on supplements and other remedies and ask about how to safely use these together with your drug treatments.

Doctors will be concerned if you want to stop taking your drug treatments and rely solely on other approaches. They'll point out that your joints are likely to deteriorate without the help of conventional medicines.

It's tempting to think that, in comparison to the powerful drug treatments used in rheumatoid arthritis, supplements and complementary remedies are natural and always safe. However, it's important to be cautious and, as with conventional medicines, ask if any research supports the use of a particular supplement or remedy for rheumatoid arthritis. Don't take anything in excess – as Pat pointed out – as this may cause problems. For example, 2 or 3 g of vitamin C a day taken on a regular basis may cause kidney stones. You might blame this problem on your conventional medicines when it may in fact be caused by taking a megadose (a dose that exceeds the recommended daily allowance) of the vitamin supplement.

Check whether or not there are any possible interactions between other remedies and supplements and your conventional medicines. It's not always clear what's in some products, so if your doctor can't help, ask a pharmacist. Whatever you do, try to keep lines of communication open between yourself and your doctor, and don't assume you're on your own if you stop taking medicines for a time. For example, it's a good idea to have regular check-ups even if you've decided against drug treatment for the moment.

Fish oils

Some people say that fish oils help, and there's some evidence to support this. The polyunsaturated fatty acids in these oils may play a part in stopping the production of the prostaglandins that cause inflammation.

There's some research that suggests the oils may indeed be beneficial. According to a report in the *Drug and Therapeutics Bulletin* (1996), in four trials fish oil supplements helped to improve symptoms such as joint tenderness and fatigue in patients with rheumatoid arthritis. In most trials, a daily 10–20-mg supplement was used.

However, the report also notes that supplements may cause mild nausea and belching and may make asthma worse in people who are sensitive to aspirin. At higher doses, the supplements may lead to a rise in blood sugar concentrations in non-insulin dependent diabetics.

A review in the *Scandinavian Journal of Rheumatology* (1999), which looked at diet and rheumatoid arthritis, concluded that, though the evidence is contradictory, fish oil does seem to have an anti-inflammatory effect, but it is weak. Also, it's not clear what the optimum daily dose should be at the moment.

Given this and the fact that it's not clear if there are any interactions between fish oil supplements and rheumatoid arthritis drugs, it may be best to incorporate the oils into your diet by, for instance, eating oil-rich fish such as mackerel, sardines or salmon at least once a week.

Ginger

This is thought to help because of its anti-inflammatory properties. However, there's no hard evidence to support its use in rheumatoid arthritis and it's unclear how much you should take.

A simple way to take ginger regularly is to make tea from it, using a couple of slices of peeled ginger root.

Selenium

This is a beneficial trace element that people with rheumatoid arthritis have reduced levels of. There's debate as to whether or not selenium supplements can relieve pain and joint inflammation. Some people think it helps, but there's no firm evidence to support this. It's unlikely to interact with rheumatoid arthritis drugs, so it may be worth a try to see if it helps you.

Glucosamine

This substance is found in healthy joints and may have a mild anti-inflammatory effect, though the evidence for this is unclear and trials have only been carried out on small numbers of people for a short time (just four to eight weeks). Also, many of the trials involved people with osteoarthritis rather than rheumatoid arthritis.

It's an expensive supplement, but is probably safe to take with conventional drugs. More research is needed to find out about its benefits and risks.

Echinacea

The extract from this wild flower is reputed to stimulate the immune system, and there's some evidence to support this. Some people take it at the first sign of illness, such as when they feel they're coming down with a cold, and to generally boost their immune system.

It's unclear whether or not echinacea interacts with any of the drugs used to treat rheumatoid arthritis, but, if you're looking to boost your immune system because you keep falling ill, be careful. If you're taking steroids or a DMARD, rather than taking echinacea you should get your white blood count checked if you're succumbing repeatedly to infections, unexplained fevers or nasty sore throats or find it's taking you a long time to recover from an illness. As discussed in previous chapters, certain drugs affect your immune system. You therefore need to tell your doctor what's happening because your drug treatment may need to be changed and this may be enough to solve the problem.

Immune suppressants

If a product is described as an 'immune suppressant', check with your doctor if it's safe to take this. Thunder god vine, for example, which is widely used in Chinese medicine as a treatment for rheumatoid arthritis, is a powerful immunosuppressant and so it should only be taken under careful supervision.

Green-lipped mussel extract

This is reputedly good for osteoarthritis, but it's unclear whether or not it's helpful for rheumatoid arthritis. Also, there's little information about whether or not it interacts with conventional medicines. Your doctor or pharmacist might be prepared to research whether or not the active ingredient in the extract interacts with other medicines.

Evening primrose oil

This oil contains the anti-inflammatory substance gamma-linoleic acid, which seems to promote the beneficial prostaglandins as opposed to the ones that have unwanted side-effects (discussed, in particular, in Chapter 6, under the heading New NSAIDs).

As we saw earlier, Pat thinks evening primrose oil helps her, but research trials so far have provided contradictory evidence about its value for rheumatoid arthritis. Again, more research is needed to find out whether or not it's useful and what dose you should take.

St John's wort

Some people take this herb – commonly called the 'sunshine herb' – if they're feeling depressed. Research so far into this plant seems to show that it works as well as conventional drugs for the treatment of mild to moderate depression, but more research is needed into its possible long-term effects – don't assume there are none.

There have been reports that St John's wort may cause eye damage in sunlight and be linked to cataracts. However, these reports may not be that relevant in this case as the research involved looking at the effects of huge doses of just one of the plant's active ingredients on calves' lenses in a laboratory setting.

More importantly, the Department of Health issued advice in 2000 about how St John's wort may prevent some prescription medicines from working properly. This list includes cyclosporin, warfarin, digoxin, theophylline (used to treat asthma and chronic bronchitis), some antidepressants and oral contraceptives. Further, it advised that you should consult your doctor if you've been taking the herb together with any of these prescription medicines. You shouldn't suddenly stop taking the herb, though, because the dose of your prescription medicine might first have to be changed depending on which drug you're taking.

Noni juice

This comes from a tree found in French Polynesia and it's claimed that the juice has anti-inflammatory properties, can boost the immune system and has no side-effects. However, it's an expensive juice and there's no hard evidence that it works.

Complementary therapies

It is possible to self-treat with herbal and homeopathic remedies bought from pharmacies and health shops, but it's best to see a trained therapist – say, a medical herbalist – to make sure you're getting the best and safest treatment. Double-check with your herbalist, but herbs shouldn't normally be taken if you're pregnant or breastfeeding.

Whatever type of therapist you see, make sure they are qualified and happy to answer your questions. Find out from your GP if they can refer you to a therapist on the NHS. If you can only get private treatment, check in advance how much it'll cost and how many sessions you'll need.

Beware of anyone who is defensive about their training, unhappy to answer your questions or promises a cure-all. Also steer clear of someone who isn't happy to work alongside your doctor or advises you to stop taking your prescription drugs.

General points about diet

Aim for a varied, wholesome diet with at least five portions of fruit and vegetables a day. Avoid refined foods, choosing instead wholemeal bread and so on as these contain a larger number of micronutrients, which it's important to have. Try to have some fish each week, too.

The question of whether or not you need to take additional vitamin and/or mineral supplements is best answered by talking to your doctor and a dietitian if necessary. Calcium and occasionally vitamin D supplements may be advised, to keep your bones healthy, but your doctor will tell you how much you can safely take. Also, ask your doctor about whether or not a vitamin E supplement or a diet rich in vitamin E might be helpful. Vitamin E is known to be an antioxidant because it lessens the damage caused by molecules produced by the body called free radicals. Some research has found that a daily 1.2-g dose had a mild painkilling effect in the body, though a lot more work needs to be done in this area.

As mentioned earlier, you need to be cautious about self-treating with higher doses of any one vitamin or mineral because of possible side-effects. A standard multivitamin supplement should be fine, though.

It's worth getting your doctor's views on whether or not a low-fat vegetarian diet could be of benefit, as some people find this helps. Make sure you get the help of a dietitian before you do try this out so that you can ensure you achieve an interesting balanced diet.

There's been some research into fasting for short periods, but no good evidence exists at the moment that this is a safe, beneficial thing to do.

Non-prescription medicines

Don't forget that medicines such as hayfever remedies or cough suppressants could possibly interact with your other drugs, so check all information leaflets very carefully. If in doubt, always ask the pharmacist if there is any interaction between other medicines such as these and your rheumatoid arthritis drugs.

Further Reading

The British Medical Association (1997) *BMA New Guide to Medicines & Drugs*, Dorling Kindersley.

Drug and Therapeutics Bulletin, 34 (8), August 1996.

Drug and Therapeutics Bulletin, 36 (1), January 1998.

Jawad, Ali S. M. (1996) *Rheumatoid Arthritis: A Patient's Guide*, Martin Dunitz.

Rowlands, Barbara (1997) *The* Which? *Guide to Complementary Medicine, Which?* Books.

Scandinavian Journal of Rheumatology, 28, 1999, pp. 201–9.

Useful Addresses

Arthritis Research Campaign
St Mary's Court
St Mary's Gate
Chesterfield
Derbyshire S41 7TD
Tel: 01246 558033
Website: www.arc.org.uk

Arthritis Care
18 Stephenson Way
London NW1 2HD
Helpline: 020 7380 6555
Website: www.arthritiscare.org.uk

Arthritis National Research Foundation
200 Oceangate
Suite 440
Long Beach
California
CA 90802
Fax: 00 1 562 983 1410
Website: www.curearthritis.org

British Sjogren's Syndrome Association
Unit 1
Manor Workshops
West End
Nailsea
Bristol BS48 4DD
Tel: 01275 854215
Website: www.BSSassociation@compuserve.com

Digestive Disorders Foundation
3 St Andrews Place
London NW1 4LB
Tel: 020 7486 0341
Website: www.digestivedisorders.org.uk

NHS Direct
Tel: 0845 4647
Website: www.nhsdirect.nhs.uk

NHS Health Information, First Health Information Service
Tel: 0800 665544

National Institute of Medical Herbalists
56 Longbrook Street
Exeter
Devon EX4 6AH
Tel: 01392 426022
Website: www.btinternet.com/~nimh

National Osteoporosis Society
PO Box 10
Radstock
Bath BA3 3YB
Tel: 01761 471771
Helpline: 01761 472721
Website: www.nos.org.uk

Index

alcohol: DMARDs 37, 40, 44, 50, 52, 55, 58, 60; NSAIDs 29; steroids 75
anaemia 4
analgesics 10, 21–3; side-effects 22–3; types 21
azathioprine (Imuran) 50–2; side-effects 51

biological agents 76–9
bone marrow stem cell transplants 82

celecoxib (Celebrex) 79, 80
chickenpox and steroids 72
children 2; drugs 19
Chlorambucil 60–1
collagen 82
complementary therapies 86–8, 92
corticosteroids *see* steroids
Cyclophosphamide 58–60, 66; side-effects 59
Cyclosporin 55–8; side-effects 56–7

depression 18
diabetes 69, 72
diet 5, 92–3
disease-modifying anti-rheumatic drugs (DMARDs) 10–11, 30; azathioprine (Imuran) 50–2;

Chlorambucil 60–1; combination therapy 61–2; course of treatment 32; Cyclophosphamide 58–60; Cyclosporin 55–8; early treatment 30–1; Enbrel 76–8; gold 44–7; hydroxychloroquine 47–50; Leflunomide (Arava) 40–4; methotrexate 32–7; Penicillamine (Distamine) 53–5; Remicade 76, 78–9; side-effects 14; sulphasalazine 37–40; types 31–2
doctors: 12-13; diagnosis 5–8
drugs: contraception 18; finding information 12–14; for flare-ups 18–19; interactions 15; names of 16; new 76–80; non-prescription 93; pregnancy and breastfeeding 16–17; safety checks 16; side-effects 14–15; step-up dose 14; taking part in trials 83–5; types used 10–11; unexpected effects 15

echinacea 90
Enbrel 76–8
'erosions' 7–8
etodolac (Lodine) 79
evening primrose oil 91

fertility 18; DMARDs 36, 40, 43, 46, 52, 58, 60
fish oils 88–9

ginger 89
glucosamine 90
gold (Myochrisin) 44–7; monitoring 45; side-effects 45
green-lipped mussel extract 90–1

heart problems 28
holidays 19
homeopathy 87
hormone replacement therapy 20
hormones 5
hydrocortisone 68
hydroxychloroquine (Plaquenil) 47–50; monitoring 49; side-effects 48

immune suppressants: supplements 90. *See also* DMARDs
inheritance 5

Leflunomide (Arava) 40–4; monitoring 42–3; side-effects 41–2
lymphoma 14

meloxicam (Mobic) 79
methotrexate 31–2, 36–7; monitoring 35; and other drugs 34–5; pregnancy and breastfeeding 36; side-effects 33–4
Methylprednisolone 66, 68

monoclonal antibodies 83

nodules: from methotrexate 34, 61; rheumatoid 3
non-steroidal anti-inflammatory drugs (NSAIDs) 10; new 79–80; with other medicines 28; side-effects 25–8; taking 24–5; types 23–4; who should avoid 28–9
noni juice 92

osteoporosis 20, 70, 71

painkillers *see* analgesics
Penicillamine (Distamine) 53–5; side-effects 53–4
prednisolone 68
pregnancy and breastfeeding: analgesics 23; DMARDs 36, 38, 43, 46, 49–50, 52, 55, 57, 60; drugs 16–17; NSAIDs 29; steroids 73
Prosorba column 80–1

Remicade 76, 78–9
rheumatoid arthritis: causes 5; defined 1–2; diagnosis 5–8; severity and prognosis 8–9; symptoms 3–4; who is affected 2
rofecoxib (Vioxx) 79, 80

St John's wort 91
selenium 89
sex life: drugs 18
Sjogren's syndrome 4, 15; and sex 18
steroids 11; action and use 63–5; injections 66–9;

minimizing the effects of 71–2; monitoring 74; side-effects 15, 69–70; tablet form 65–6; who can take 70–1
stomach ulcers: drug side-effect 25–7
stroke 28
sulphasalazine (Salazopyrin EN) 37–40; side-effects 38–9
supplements 86–92

therapies, non-drug: bone

marrow stem cell transplants 82; collagen 82; monoclonal antibodies 83; Prosorba column 80–1
treatments: see diet; drugs; surgical procedures
triamcinolone 68

vaccinations 19; DMARDs 40, 43, 50, 52, 55, 58, 60; steroids 75
vitamins 92–3

warfarin 67